Advance Praise for
Transformed by Postpartum Depression

Dr. Walker Ladd has forged the future for maternal mental health. Her provocative book, Transformed by Postpartum Depression, *will challenge and change clinicians, researchers, and the public. Finally, the paradigm of PPD has been broadened to include trauma and the human condition. She has exposed a missing piece of the postpartum puzzle. Thank you, Walker!*

—**Jane Honikman,** MA, Founder,
Postpartum Support International

Walker Ladd has achieved greatness in the PPD community with her emphasis on trauma, transformation, and personal growth. What makes Transformed by Postpartum Depression *so uniquely powerful is that Ladd stands in the face of preconceived notions and challenges them with the stories and voices of real women who speak the truth and deserve to be heard. The conviction of these experiences holds tremendous healing power on behalf of the PPD woman seeking support as well as valued wisdom for the clinician who is accompanying this journey.*

—**Karen Kleiman,** MSW, Founder & Director,
The Postpartum Stress Center; Author,
Therapy and the Postpartum Woman

I found Walker Ladd's book an intelligent analysis of the debilitating process of postpartum depression and the significant impact it had on the lives of women and those close to them. It was sensitively written with elements of intense sympathy, empathy, and consideration for the courageous narratives which permeate throughout the book. Powerful personal thoughts were shared on the helplessness of suicidality and the need for something more than the superficiality of talk, but instead about the need for a solution and the hope that they would eventually improve. Walker's book offers a specific insight into the plight of mothers who have suffered from postpartum depression, and the cathartic, emotional journey they had to take to seek the peace they deserved. I really enjoyed reading the book and found it captured the elements of PPD in a very interesting and sensitive fashion.

Dr Jane Hanley, Past President of the International Marcé Society for Perinatal Mental Health, Hon Senior Lec- turer in Primary Care, Public and Mental Health, College of Human and Health Sciences, Swansea University, Swansea, Wales

Praeclarus Press, LLC

2504 Sweetgum Lane

Amarillo, Texas 79124 USA

806-367-9950

www.PraeclarusPress.com

DISCLAIMER

The information contained in this publication is advisory only and is not intended to replace sound clinical judgment or individualized patient care. The author disclaims all warranties, whether expressed or implied, including any warranty as the quality, accuracy, safety, or suitability of this information for any particular purpose.

ISBN: 978-1-946665-41-6

Cover Design: Ken Tackett and Walker Ladd

Back Page Design: Walker Ladd

Developmental Editing: Kathleen Kendall-Tackett

Copyediting: Chris Tackett

Layout & Design: Nelly Murariu

Transformed by Postpartum Depression

Women's Stories of Trauma and Growth

SECOND EDITION

Walker Ladd, PhD

Praeclarus Press, LLC

www.PraeclarusPress.com

Men say they know many things;
But lo! they have taken wings, —
The arts and sciences,
And a thousand appliances;
The wind that blows
Is all that anybody knows.

– THOREAU –

For my sister, Sara

ACKNOWLEDGMENTS

I would like to acknowledge the extraordinary women who have shared their stories with me over the years, and Jane Honikman, for your vision, friendship, and guts.

And to Gwen, thank you for helping me stay.

TABLE OF CONTENTS

FOREWORD

– Sarah Brumpton –

Founder: Open House Nottingham, UKIn early 2011,
I read the first edition of *Transformed by Postpartum
Depression* approximately eighteen months after my
discharge from the Dr. Margaret Oates Mother and
Baby Unit (MBU), which at that time was located at the
Queens Medical Centre in Nottingham, England.

I was hospitalized for eight weeks while being treated for severe postnatal depression with mild psychotic features following the birth of my second son. As the name implies, the MBU is an inpatient perinatal psychiatric ward for mothers with a serious mental illness and their babies. The philosophy of the unit is to treat and care about mothers while promoting the mother/baby relationship.

Those eight weeks were the start of my recovery from an illness that had started some months beforehand. For my family and me, it was one of the most traumatic experiences we have ever been through, and to this day, I find it hard to think about what would have happened if I were not admitted. My treatment involved a number of medication combinations until the right combination was found. For me, the MBU was, and still is, a place of hope and recovery. I was fortunate to be fully discharged from the Perinatal Psychiatry Service soon after leaving the hospital and was keen to use my experience to support others in a similar situation. That desire led me to Walker's unique first book.

The remarkable women in *Transformed by Postpartum Depression* described a strength to keep going in the face of life-threatening illness, fear, isolation, and trauma. While living on different

1

continents, I was struck by how I could fully appreciate the emotions of each of them. I found myself in tears more than once, yet I was able to draw on their courage and motivation as I learned how they were transformed by their experiences.

I feel compelled to mention the differences in the healthcare systems between the US and the UK. I was in complete awe of the women and their families who had to navigate the insurance system and source their own specialist healthcare professionals while desperately trying to get through each day and care for their babies. There certainly were times when I thought that added to the trauma experienced.

There were fifteen MBUs at the time of my admittance to the hospital following significant investment; this has since increased by four. Additionally, every National Health Service local delivery area has a Perinatal Community Mental Health Service. The Nottingham MBU has also relocated to a new purpose-built facility.

I'm in no doubt that none of this would have been possible without the incredible work of Dr. Margaret Oates. Dr. Oates was a formidable leading light in the establishment of perinatal psychiatry as a subsection of psychiatry in the UK and beyond. She was awarded a lifetime achievement award from the Royal College of Psychiatrists in 2013.

I did go on to use my experience positively through the establishment of a small charity called Open House Nottingham which I co-founded with another former MBU patient who has since qualified as a therapist. I have delivered talks to healthcare professionals, charities, and students focused on my lived experience. Some of my proudest moments have been when I witness women supporting each other at our three peer support groups or when individuals share their experiences at a time when they are at their most vulnerable. I've also gained friends for life. One thing that has become clear to me through my work with

Open House Nottingham is that while women may be diagnosed with the same illness/condition, no two women will experience them the same, and that's key when it comes to supporting those women. They need to be heard as individuals.

I'm grateful to Walker for her dedication to her research into perinatal mood and anxiety disorders, which goes beyond the clinical symptoms, prevalence, and statistics, allowing those with lived experience to see beyond them and recognize that they too can be positively changed by them.

FOREWORD

– Ivy Shih Leung –

Author, *One mom's journey to motherhood: Infertility, childbirth complications, and postpartum depression, Oh My!*

PPD was a major turning point in my life. Before PPD, my life was one bumpy road going in no particular direction. I lacked self-confidence. After PPD, I read about numerous books and articles about maternal mental health disorders, published a book, blogged, provided phone and email support to other mothers, and volunteered for and befriended numerous Postpartum Support International (PSI) members around the country. I gained a voice. I gained self-confidence at work and in my daily life and activities. It was the absence of books by PPD survivors that prompted me to write my own book, which I started writing during my PPD recovery. It was published in 2011. My PPD journey represents a tiny segment of my entire life, but it had the greatest impact. PPD was a necessary step in transforming me into the person I am today. I was honored to be a participant in the first edition of *Transformed by Postpartum Depression*. I am deeply honored that Walker has come full circle to ask me to write a foreword for this new edition.

I remember when I received a copy of the first edition of *Transformed by Postpartum Depression* in December 2014. I was beyond thrilled for Walker. Her years of interviews, research, writing, and editing had blossomed into an important book that gives voice to these women whose words describing their thoughts, feelings, and experiences needed to be shared with other women, their families, and mental/medical health practitioners.

5

Transformed by Postpartum Depression differs from any other book ever published about PPD. It presents the stories of twenty-five PPD survivors and how their individual experiences transformed and empowered them. This is an important book for women suffering from PPD because they need to see that other women like themselves not only survived but were able to use their experiences to become stronger than ever before and to use their strength to make better lives for themselves.

This book is also important for all individuals in the medical and mental health occupations who need to treat expectant and new mothers at any given point in their careers. In fact, in my opinion, this book should be MANDATORY reading for all OB/GYNs, nurses, general practitioners, doulas, midwives, lactation consultants, psychiatrists, psychologists, and social workers.

I wish I could've found Walker's book when I was sick with PPD and was desperately seeking other people's stories but only found those written by celebrities. *Transformed by Postpartum Depression* is a critical contribution that helps shrink the size of the void of books written by PPD survivors. Walker takes the experiences of the 25 women and craftily weaves their words throughout each chapter, speaking to what PPD is, its prevalence, its risk factors, false notions about PPD and motherhood, and how untreated PPD impacted them physically and psychologically. Walker's description of how these women transformed through the trauma of untreated PPD gives women hope for recovery.

LIST OF TABLES

LIST OF FIGURES

PREFACE TO THE NEW EDITION

For we think back through our mothers if we are women.

– Virginia Woolf –

Following the birth of my daughter in 2003, I worked as a maternal mental health advocate, birth doula, and writer. Through that work, I met extraordinary women who described how postpartum depression (PPD) had changed them in powerful ways. These were women who amazed me with their stories of survival, strength, and commitment to help others, despite unimaginable pain. They had suffered—greatly. But many, if not the majority, told me that the suffering catalyzed significant personal change. This change was my interest as a researcher and became the focus of my doctoral dissertation (Karraa, 2013).

What was it about the nature of PPD to change the trajectory of a woman's life? How does a woman experience this change? What could we learn from women that might deepen our under-standing of the pathology and its meaning in women's lives? Questions like these fueled my early curiosity and inspired my writing of the first edition of *Transformed by Postpartum Depression: Women's Stories of Trauma and Growth* (Karraa, 2014).

The first edition described my grounded theory study of the transformational nature of PPD with 20 women who identified as (a) having had PPD, and (b) they were transformed by the experience. In that study, four semi-structured interview questions were used:

1. A descriptive question elicited a description of the phenomenon of transformation through postpartum

depression: *How would you describe your process of transformation through PPD?*

2. An exploratory question investigated the phenomenon of transformation through PPD: *In what ways did you experience the process of transformation through postpartum depression?*

3. An explanatory question probed for patterns, processes, or categories related to the transformation through PPD: *What were the ways you saw yourself transforming?*

4. An emancipatory question explored the evolving nature and processes of transformation through PPD: *How do you experience this transformation currently?*

Interviews with the 20 participants resulted in over 300 pages of transcribed text. Open, axial, and selective coding revealed a theoretical model of untreated PPD as traumatic, and that from trauma, women experienced traumatic growth. This process occurred through four stages: **before** postpartum depression (*I Was Unprepared*), **during** postpartum depression (*I Was Shattered*), **after** postpartum depression (*I Am a Different Person*), and **beyond** postpartum depression (*Paradox and Purpose*).

In order to triangulate the theoretical findings, I created and administered the *Changing Depression Survey* (Appendix A) from October 2013 to January 2014, obtaining data from a total of 486 respondents. When asked if PPD had been life-threatening, 61% (n = 297) responded "Yes"; 38.9% (n = 189) responded "No." Perceptions of care provider failure, and identification of self as the primary agent in seeking and obtaining treatment. The question "Who was MOST responsible for your getting help for postpartum depression (PPD)?" yielded data regarding women's perception of self as an agent in accessing care for PPD. Given six options (see Appendix A), 65.4% (n = 318) selected "Self."

Another method of triangulating the original data included peer review. I sent findings to six experts in the fields of post-traumatic growth or perinatal mood and anxiety disorders. I then interviewed them to obtain professional perspectives on the theory that PPD can be experienced as traumatic and that post-traumatic growth can occur as a result. The first edition began a dialogue on the traumatic nature of untreated PPD, the value of women's subjective experience in postpartum research, and the role providers and experts play in forming beliefs and practices regarding perinatal mood and anxiety disorders (Richmond, 2019).

NEW EDITION CHANGES

Much has changed since the first edition. For one, my name; I was divorced in 2015. My name is Walker Ladd, and this new edition will be correctly cited. Secondly, the previous foreword needed to be updated to reflect an evolution in readership. The new foreword written by both Sarah Brumpton and Ivy Shih-Leung offers readers an invitation to the book that is grounded in personal and professional experiences with perinatal mood and anxiety disorders. Lastly, and most importantly, I wanted to revisit the theory of the transformative nature of PPD from an evolved perspective based on my curiosity as a researcher about the nature of change itself:

- What has changed in how women experience PPD as traumatic?

- What has changed in the research about PPD?

- What has changed in social constructs of postpartum depression among experts in the field?

- What would happen to the theory if I talked about my own experience with PPD? More accurately, how could I not share?

To answer these questions, I conducted new five interviews with using the same interview questions and format in order to see if there were changes in the lived experience. Second, I reviewed the current research in the prevalence, risk factors, and effects of PPD. Third, I sought additional professional perspectives from additional leaders in the field regarding the traumatic nature of untreated PPD. Fourth, I wrote about my own experience.

Positivist research lays claim to unbiased truth, attempting to remove the researcher from the research as if we could discover a truth that could be objectively identified by anyone looking at it. Definitions of things are then categorized and cross-referenced— and new phenomena are tested against those hard truths. A rock, for example, has certain observable properties in matter and form.

In many circumstances, this approach is necessary to gain the cleanest, clearest results, such as in a double-blind experiment of a new clinical drug. I am respectful of and grateful for the scientific method and its tenacity in pursuing the truth. However, my paradigm as a researcher and writer is not positivist; it is interpretivist, rooted in hermeneutic phenomenology, and grounded in continental existential philosophy.

From this position, I reject the notion that objective truth is inherently real or measurable but rather, constructed by multiple entities, including society, culture, history, and individuals, and co-existing with objective reality. Ongoing work in the field of quantum physics supports the notion that objective reality does not exist but instead, is constructed in multiple ways (Proietti et al., 2019).

From this ontological perspective, the reality of PPD cannot be known, defined, nor quantified. By definition, it is constructed in real-time, every time, in multiple ways by multiple people. I take the position that the reality of PPD is co-constructed in a dynamic and changing fashion that cannot be observed as only one thing.

Context provides a common language for communication about PPD, namely the systems of knowledge that have named it thus far: medical science, psychology, psychiatry, and the historical and social contexts of all of those bodies of knowledge come with the language. Think about it; I can write three letters in "PPD," and the construct of the disorder is understood by the reader. In the UK, the letters would be "PND" for postnatal depression.

I argue that the meaning we make of the idea (construct) of what we call, "postpartum depression", is created through our historical, social, and cultural relation to it—evidenced by the words and letters we use to describe it. Researchers describe postpartum depression in the scientific literature using the language of positivism. Mental health scholars and practitioners describe postpartum depression from a therapeutic perspective using psychological clinical language. Bloggers know PPD as something they have lived and write about it in personal language. In the United Kingdom, it is called postnatal depression, or PND. In each circumstance, the language reflects the different ways the experience exists.

Doctors, researchers, therapists, women, men—past, present, and future use the language agreed upon to communicate an experience of PPD. Yet, how effective is this arrangement?

Hermeneutic phenomenological philosopher Martin Heidegger argued that the essence of human understanding comes in the shape of language. Language is the "house of being." The language, the words we use to communicate with one another, houses the potential for interpretation of the significance of the experience.

From traditional positivist paradigms of empirical science, women experiencing a perinatal mood or anxiety disorder only by using that language—the language of medicine and science "postpartum depression". From a hermeneutic phenomenological perspective, language not only conveys *what* PPD is, but *how* it is. Hermeneutic phenomenology reveals the nature of experience through circular examination of the parts involved in co-constructing the whole. Applied to qualitative research, this cyclical process positions the researcher as one of the parts. Hermeneutic phenomenological research methods, boldly transparent, acknowledge that the researcher cannot possibly be objective, bracketing aside all biases. Even the words used to identify what they are studying are embedded within their educational history, cultural context, and socially designed significance. My use of the term PPD comes with all of the history of the word, the history of how I learned it, taught to use it, and my interpretation of it in my own experience with it.

So, what is to be studied about PPD? Everything. Ultimately, women's experience, the perspectives of the professionals and scientific community, the historical and social contexts, and my own experience are parts of the whole. Therefore, I am sharing my own experience with PPD in this second edition to hopefully give a fuller, more authentic, and transparent experience of the nature of PPD to you, the reader, and your own experience with PPD. Paradigm Shift: Our Stories

Your perspective and interpretation of the experiences shared in this book are parts of a future understanding of the significance of this event on the lives of women. Unfortunately, maternal mental illness holds a unique place in the minds of society. The pairing of constructs of motherhood with constructs of madness remains the most powerful and profoundly rooted stigma in society's collective psyche: mentally ill mothers are dangerous and potentially violent. Generations of women have endured unnecessary suffering as a result of these stigmatizing assumptions, prejudicial attitudes, and discriminatory actions about mothers with depression and anxiety.

My mother had major depression for most of her adult life, including severe postpartum depression after having me. She spent the last part of her life treated for depression by her oncologist. My mom spent a lifetime suffering from and through depression. She was ignored, told it was in her head, overmedicated, undermedicated. Her depression was ultimately invisible to the medical establishment, only to face the end of her life just as invisible. She passed in 2010, at home, a few months before I started my doctoral program. In my darkest moments of depression, I feel her presence with me.

More recently, my sister had major surgery following a cancer diagnosis at age 56. Intensive care and no food by mouth was the expected recovery protocol. When she was diagnosed, she had been treated successfully for depression with an SSRI for over 20 years. Her surgeon, an expert in the surgical procedure, and the entire pre-op staff at this leading university hospital knew that this medication was on her chart. They knew that she would not be able to take any food or water by mouth for a minimum of two days due to the post-operative feeding tube, and yet, they did not tell her to titrate down before the procedure. Did they not know that patients suffer horrible discontinuity syndrome if they cannot swallow their medication? There were no psychiatrists on daily rounds. At day three, we brought it to the attention of the physical therapist and asked for a psych consult. The psychiatrists confirmed discontinuity syndrome but could only treat the symptoms (nightmares, dizziness) because the SSRI was not manufactured in liquid form so it could not be administered through IV.

Part of the recovery in this oncology post-op unit included visits from pets, but no psychiatrist nor a licensed mental health-care provider. No one on that unit was visited by a psychiatric provider. Just pets. My sister's suffering was 100% preventable, as is the case with perinatal mood or anxiety disorders that or during end-of-life care.

The suffering described by the women in this book was also preventable. PPD was not the major cause of suffering; untreated PPD was. The 25 women interviewed for this book, and the majority of the 486 women who completed the Changing Depression Survey, did not receive preventive care, nor were they treated before the symptoms were severe, nor with accurate treatments to help them avoid the worst suffering they had ever imagined. They survived through their own means, but barely. Loving, strong, smart, creative women who were deconstructed by the onset of a perinatal mood or anxiety disorder, found a way back, found a way to stay alive, and realize a sense of purpose and fulfillment of personal potential.

DESCRIPTION OF BOOK

The second edition is divided into two parts.

Part I: Understanding Untreated Postpartum Depression begins with a new introduction where I share my own experience with untreated PPD following the birth of my son, Ziggy. I also introduce the 25 women who participated in this book project.

Chapter 1: Understanding Untreated Postpartum Depression reviews current clinical definitions, screening instruments and practices, and research regarding prevalence, risk factors, and the effects of PPD on women and children.

Chapter 2: Before Postpartum Depression: I Was Unprepared describes the first dimension of the transformational process through PPD as women reported being unprepared for the onset of symptoms.

Chapter 3: During Postpartum Depression: I Was Shattered describes the traumatic impact of untreated symptoms of PPD.

Chapter 4: Running the Gauntlet: Provider Failure and Getting Better reveals the tragic failure of providers to address, treat, or acknowledge the symptoms of PPD and the extraordinary ways women worked to find the help they critically needed.

Chapter 5: After Postpartum Depression: I Am a Different Person describes how women experienced the transformation in their lives, relationships, and professional interests.

Chapter 6: Beyond Postpartum Depression: Paradox and Purpose explains how women experienced transformative growth in the final dimension—where levels of growth surpassed resiliency or recovery.

Part II: Theoretical and Professional Perspectives begins with *Chapter 7: Trauma and Transformation* reviewing theories of change and growth through adversity in order to home in on the most accurate understanding of the trauma and transformation of PPD.

Chapter 8: Professional Perspectives, presents interviews conducted with five experts in the field: Cheryl Beck, Jane Shakespeare-Finch, Karen Kleiman, Pec Indman, and Jane Honikman. The variety of expertise and opinion of the construct of PPD as a traumatic life event is both disparate and thought-provoking.

Finally, *Chapter 9: When PPD Grows Up: New Reflections and Future Directions* concludes the book by circling back to the current view of PPD and the expanding conversation and paradigm offered in this book and describing future inquiry into the experience of perinatal mood and anxiety disorders over the lifespan.

I am grateful for the opportunity to revisit this book with the fresh eyes of hindsight. So, we begin where I started this journey 20 years ago, in Seattle.

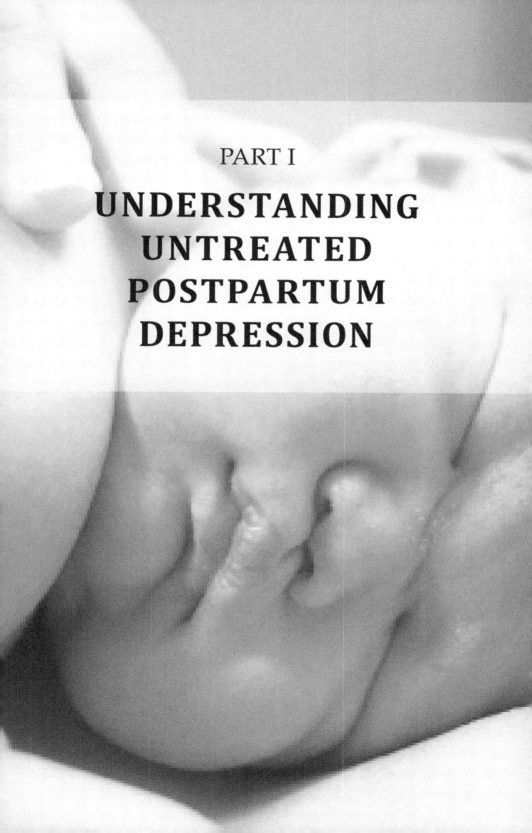

PART I

UNDERSTANDING UNTREATED POSTPARTUM DEPRESSION

INTRODUCTION:
"I'M READY, MOM"

My family has a grand tradition. After a woman
gives birth, she goes mad.
– Adrienne Martini, Hillbilly Gothic –

G reen Lake is a man-made lake in the middle of Seattle, Washington. It is about 3 miles around and gorgeous. When I moved to Seattle to attend graduate school, I fell in love with it. I went nearly every day. One day, making my way around Green Lake, I heard a little boy say, "I'm ready, Mom." He sounded school age, maybe 7 or 8. I turned around, looking over my right shoulder, expecting to see a mom and son getting ready to pass me on bikes. There was no one there. A month later, I was pregnant with Ziggy.

The first two home pregnancy tests were negative. I went to see my family practitioner for a blood test. Sobbing while the nurse did the blood draw, I knew I was pregnant, but maybe science would prove me wrong. I was at my internship office when they called to confirm the pregnancy—with an estimated due date of 11/15/00.

At 8 weeks, I was at my internship and started bleeding. My clinical supervisor, who would share some choice words with me later in my journey, looked at me with a sad face and said, "These things happen, Walker." Fear, as I had never known, filled my heart. I called my doctor, and she told me to go to the hospital immediately. My husband was working. I drove myself to the hospital for an ultrasound. I was terrified and alone.

21

But there he was: Ziggy. The same creature I had heard at the lake, the same creature I knew was in my belly when I stared at negative pregnancy tests, there he was. Healthy. I remember crying so hard that the tech told me not to drive home. I had proven science and my doomsday supervisor wrong. I drove myself home and didn't look back on any worries regarding the "viability" of my boy.

BEFORE POSTPARTUM DEPRESSION

The pregnancy continued with no further incidents. I exercised, ate right, and planned for the big day. The doctor started saying Ziggy was "big" late into my second trimester. When a medical provider tells you that the baby is big, you have been assigned to the c-section queue lurking in the back of the doc's mind. I was 10 days past my estimated due date, and the next day was going to be induced, when around midnight, labor started. I called my doula and tried to rest.

I remember the feel of my grandfather's dresser under my hands as I steadied myself to get dressed. I wore a black cardigan sweater, blue t-shirt, and black maternity pants from K-Mart. Six days later, they would be bagged up and handed to me like forensic evidence of what had gone down. What had been killed. Blood soaked underwear, puke stained shirt. How did I ever get them off of me? Who took them off? How did anyone keep track of them? Why do I want them back? How am I going to get them clean?

I remember walking across the street to the hospital with my husband. Seattle in November, freezing cold and wet. I was still good, still in love with my husband, still believing I was going to be okay. The last image of my marriage as I had known it was my husband walking me across the street to the hospital emergency room. It was a normal birth. I was a healthy woman. I had a healthy baby. I loved my husband, and I loved my baby.

Everything was going great. I was okay. I was birthing the son I loved more than anything I had known. My dear Ziggy, my sweet boy. More pain came, and more still. Hours of self-imposed torture because I wanted to do it "the right way," staring into the blue eyes of my doula, determined to have a natural birth. I was not prepared for what was to come.

Medical interventions to augment labor and measure the efficacy of my uterus slowly worked their way into my midbrain, the limbic system, where childhood patterns of fight, flight, or freeze kicked in: cervical checks, intrauterine catheters, Pitocin drip, more cervical checks. Pitocin with no epidural is no party. The level of pain was beyond me, but it worked to force my cervix to 10 centimeters.

I felt a sense of bearing down but started passing out in between contractions. Labor slowed. Years later, my husband told me he saw me dissociate entirely during that time, hanging on a birth bar with what felt like endless cords and tubes coming out of my vagina. He saw me leave, split off from the world.

Within the hour, and another cervical check, they told us Ziggy was stuck in my pelvis, and the call was made for a cesarean based on Ziggy's heart rate fluctuations during contractions. I remember the anesthesiologist coming into the OR prep room and putting his feet up on my hospital tray. I remember his rainbow tie-dye surgical hat and enormous mustache. I remember that he told me the epidural wouldn't hurt and would work. He lied. It hurt like hell.

They wheeled me into the operating room; I remember seeing the nurses hoisting my naked pregnant body from my hospital bed onto the surgical table, like a dead whale ready to be fileted.

The anesthesiologist took out a safety pin from the pocket of his scrubs and started poking my chest and down my body, asking me to tell him when I no longer felt the pain. I still felt it all the way down. I felt them prep me for surgery.

Trying to tell the anesthesiologist that I was feeling the prep, the OB/GYN who would perform the c-section walked in while yawning. "Why don't you have latte before opening me up?" I shouted across the room. My husband, silently mortified, patted my strapped-down arm. The OB proceeded to brag about how she had watched her own c-section and that it was no big deal. Well, Dr. Latte, it *was* a big deal. I felt you and your staff start the incision on my right side: pressure and burning, I thought they were cauterizing me—trying to make rational sense of what I was feeling. Searing heat turned to stabbing pain. The last thing I remember is trying to tell the voices behind the blue sheet brushing up against my cheek that I could feel what they were doing. Eventually, the anesthesiologist gave me so much medication that I could not feel my legs for the next two days.

Ziggy was born on 11/27/00, the same day and same hospital as Jimmy Hendrix. He was a healthy 7lbs; no big baby. Recovery was hard. I couldn't walk for the first 48 hours due to the botched epidural. The hospital kept Ziggy in the room with me, and each and every noise he made jolted me into high alert and back to the breast he went. The constant worry about milk production and tracking how long he would feed on which breast was exhausting. Nothing like being told you are 100% responsible for sustaining the life of the infant angel you had just birthed. No pressure.

I didn't sleep. I would start to doze and then startle awake, feeling like I was having another contraction. Eventually, I was able to walk and pushed Ziggy around the maternity ward in the plastic layette. My God, I loved him.

Before leaving the hospital, the nurses taught us how to put Ziggy in the car seat, how to clean his umbilical cord, and how to watch for jaundice. We were and given complimentary diapers, coupons for formula, and a plastic bag containing the black cardigan, K-Mart maternity pants, and blue t-shirt I was wearing when I was admitted.

DURING POSTPARTUM DEPRESSION

My husband and I spent the next two months muscling through, but in hindsight, we were falling apart and isolated. Having relocated to Seattle for graduate studies in clinical psychology, we had no family, no friends, no support systems near us. Seattle in late November is cold and dark. It was just the three of us.

Brain Offline

It is surreal to know the brain has shut down. Like a cutting of permanent wires, my brain was offline. Normal and vital functioning was impaired. I think the first symptom of PPD that I recognized in the category of "not right" was a pain in my hands. My wrists and fingers constantly ached. I lost my appetite in a way that I had never experienced. It was as if I could not create the sensation of hunger or taste. The food was tasteless. Eating was removed from the sensation of hunger or taste. Again, it was as if my brain was offline, as if I had swimmer's ear and maybe could just shake my head and wait it out and things would clear, that my brain would suddenly reboot. It didn't.

Around six weeks postpartum, Ziggy started sleeping through the night. I did not. When he slept on my chest, my mind raced. I would slide him over to my husband and try to sleep on the living room floor, but I was still awake. I stayed awake for the next three weeks. My primary care provider told me to drink milk at night. I stayed awake. She told me to take 50 mg of Benadryl. I stayed awake. At my six-week checkup, she prescribed Paxil. I had a horrible reaction to it and stayed awake. One of the strongest memories of my PPD is that I believed I had lost my ability to sleep. The cycle of anxiety was beginning in the early evening, becoming a night of panic attacks, spiraled into my belief that (a) I had broken my ability to sleep, and it could not be fixed, and (b) Ziggy would be better off without me.

Aurora Bridge

No sleep for one week, two weeks, then three weeks. I started spending the night on the living room floor: night after night on that floor. When I heard Zig wake up, I went in and fed him, then headed back out to the living room floor where I didn't sleep.

One night, around Christmas, I decided it would never end, that I would never be able to sleep, that my precious son didn't deserve to have such a defective mother and to jump off of the Aurora Bridge near our house. I had already contemplated suicide many times by then but had not attempted. But that night, as a marathon of the movie *A Christmas Story* played over and over, I wanted it to end. I got in my car. We didn't live that far from the bridge. It was so dark that night, and icy too. I kept trying to figure out how I could stop on the side of the road and jump without hurting the drivers in the cars behind me. It was not their fault I wanted to die.

In the Queen Anne neighborhood of Seattle, there is an on-ramp that comes off of a curvy residential street. I drove on to the bridge and put my hazards on. I wanted it over so badly. I couldn't hurt anymore. I couldn't do it one more minute. I kept driving to the other side of the bridge, hazard lights on, circling around, and trying it again. I never stopped. I eventually drove home and got back on the living room floor. No one ever knew I had left. I said nothing the next day. The thoughts of suicide were constant. I thought about the times my own father attempted suicide and failed, and was ashamed that I was like him, having gone that far in trying but failing.

Later the next day, I was standing behind my husband while he was changing Ziggy's diapers, when I passed out from exhaustion. Throughout my PPD, my husband kept telling me that I just needed to change my mind, that it was all under my control. "Just change your mind," was his mantra. At the time, he meant that he believed I could stop suffering through my own volition, by just changing my mind. The implication was that it was metaphorically all in my head, and that I was failing at fixing it.

He didn't understand, not sure he does to this day, and I don't blame him. What he didn't know was that my mind, the organic brain matter inside of my skull, and the negative space between synapses--definitely needed changing through medical intervention. He was suffering his own battle with anxiety and fear. He has since shared with me that my passing out that day was as scared as he had ever been.

Nonetheless, the message I got from him was that these physical symptoms were the result of my personal choice. In other words, if I fixed my own thinking, rearranged my own thoughts, I would suddenly sleep like a baby and be hungry and happy, and not want to drive to the highest bridge in Seattle and jump. This is why I didn't tell him about my driving to the Aurora Bridge when I got home that night. He wouldn't know what to do other than tell me to do something myself. I needed someone's help, not more pressure to fix myself. He wouldn't be a soft place to fall that night, nor any night to come.

Professional Lifelines

From my station on the living room floor, I called my internship supervisor and told her I was suicidal. While she had no experience with perinatal mood or anxiety disorders, and no references to share, she did say something that shook me to my core: "Walker, if you kill yourself, Ziggy will never be okay. Ever." I knew she was right.

I looked through my clinical textbooks from my graduate studies and clinical training. Two books became professional lifelines to recovery. The first, Shaila Misri's book, *Shouldn't I Be Happy: Emotional Problems of Pregnant and Postpartum Women,* had been assigned in my lifecycle course. After speaking with my supervisor that night, I scoured that book and called information for Dr. Shaila Misri's phone number in Vancouver, BC, and I left a long voice mail asking for help.

The next day, surprised that she called me back, I spoke with her on the phone, and she assured me that I could be successfully treated with the right medication. She shared, "You can't compete with chemistry," and connected me with a psychiatric nurse practitioner in Seattle. I left a voice message for the nurse practitioner, who called me back and did a short intake over the phone. She told me to either self-admit to the hospital for suicidal ideation or have someone with me 24 hours a day until I was stabilized on medication, and then she booked my appointment.

That left me with few options, unfortunately. My own mother, not very well herself, lived a few hours away by plane. When I asked if she would come, she told me she wouldn't know what to pack and didn't own a suitcase. She never did come to see Ziggy or me in Seattle. My husband's family was in Los Angeles, and stigma clouded their ability to understand a daughter-in-law with postpartum depression. My sister was in Los Angeles with three

children. My brother was in Hawaii. I needed someone immediately. I contemplated self-admission, but I could not bear the
thought of being separated from Ziggy.

I called my closest friend Gwen. Gwen had been my student
when I ran the dance program at a high school for the arts, and we
had maintained a friendship after I went on to study psychology.
She was only 21 at the time, in cooking school in Santa Barbara.
She flew into town the next day. She didn't hesitate.

Gwen went with me to my first appointment with the nurse
practitioner, who took one look at me and got samples out of her
private stash for me to take home with me. She wrote a prescription for Zoloft and Klonopin, and that night, I slept for the first
time in three weeks, and Gwen laid next to me holding my hand.
I don't think I would be alive if she hadn't helped.

ENDING PPD

Gwen stayed until I was stable. She cooked healthy meals, held
Ziggy so I could shower, did laundry, went with me to follow-up
appointments, and slept with me on the living room floor every
night, making sure I was safe and asleep. Ten days later, she went
home, and I kept looking for more understanding as to what had
happened and what to expect.

Again, I turned to research, pulling the second book from my
clinical training library, Deborah Sichel and Jeanne Driscoll's
1999 book, *Women's Moods, Women's Minds: What Every Woman
Must Know About Hormones, the Brain, and Emotional Health*. A well-
known and respected clinical psychiatric nurse and researcher,
Jeanne's details of her own experiences following the birth of
her first daughter validated my own experience and planted a
seed of wonder in the ways we talk about women's reproductive experiences. Jeanne wrote: "My transformative experience

began on April 11, 1976, with the birth of our first daughter, Lorraine" (1999, p. 3).

There was that word! **Transformative.** If someone as respected and smart as Jeanne could admit to having been changed, transformed, reshaped, reconfigured by a postpartum experience involving trauma and provider ignorance, maybe I was not alone. I devoured the writing and employed the NURSE self-care program described in *Women's Moods*: nutrition and needs, understanding, rest and relaxation, spirituality, and exercise (Sichel & Driscoll, 1999).

GETTING BETTER

The symptoms were slowly treated through medication and the NURSE program, and I continued to get better. My recovery was slow, but it was a recovery. We relocated back to Los Angeles when Ziggy was four months old, and I continued my care for PPD at my alma mater, the UCLA Women's Life Center.

My first appointment ended with the attending psychiatrist coming escorting me into the waiting room to examine Ziggy in the stroller. No one, except everyone reading this book, knows what it's like when power examines your baby. I have never been that afraid or that vulnerable. My heart stopped. If he was asleep, would she think that I was taking too much Klonopin? If he was crying, would she think that he was irritable due to the Zoloft? Would she see some evidence that I was harming the baby I loved more than life itself? We got closer, then Ziggy was awake and looked directly at the doctor with his beautiful Buddha face and smiled. She smiled, patted me on the shoulder, and whispered, "He's fine."

So, did that mean I wasn't going to be arrested? I struggled with what to make of her reassurance in the moment of tears and fear. I had worked so hard to advocate for myself and my recovery. Before that long walk through the lobby of the neuropsychiatric wing at my alma mater, I was a good mother. The moment this doctor told me she wanted to examine Ziggy, the fear of being seen as a bad mother became very real. I don't think that fear has ever left my side.

AFTER PPD

I continued treatment at the university neuropsychiatric center, cycling through residents every 6 months. Early on, I was assigned a male resident who had no idea what I was experiencing and told me to drink milk at night for insomnia. I demanded female residents, a series of young women with whom I felt safer. Then one day, I was informed that my new resident would be a man. I was a seasoned postpartum veteran by then and was NOT happy. Dr. S walked out and greeted me, looking like he had accidentally walked into the wrong waiting room. I sat down in his office and immediately asked, "What in the hell do you know about postpartum depression?" Dr. S ended up becoming my psychiatrist for the next decade.

When I got pregnant with my beautiful daughter, Miles, two years later, Dr. S was a part of a team of providers I relied on to see me through pregnancy, birth, and postpartum symptom-free. I was referred to an excellent OB/GYN who knew the science regarding SSRIs, reproductive health, and birth trauma. I got a great therapist familiar with PPD. With the teamwork of a psychiatrist, therapist, and OB/GYN, I had a happy pregnancy, birth, and postpartum period with my sweet baby girl. I *was* symptom-free, even though my OB/GYN had to tell me to bring my own Zoloft from home so that the nurses wouldn't bother me about taking it while breastfeeding. We did it, my girl and me. We did it. The four days I spent in the hospital with Miles was possibly the happiest I have ever been, even to this day.

BEYOND PPD

The fact that I had achieved such a wonderful pregnancy, birth, and postpartum through the care management of a stellar team of professionals made me determined to make meaning out of my experience with PPD. Miles was born in March. Eight months later, I was diagnosed with breast cancer. I stayed committed to maternal mental health advocacy, becoming a certified birth doula, and writing about maternal mental health research for Science and Sensibility. In 2010, I returned to school to pursue my doctoral degree in psychology.

I knew that I wanted to study postpartum depression in a way that went beyond traditional views of psychopathology. Underlying my initial wonder was a sense of human potential in women who suffer from perinatal mood or anxiety disorders. I knew that previous research had only evidenced a part of the whole experience of PPD. We have benefitted tremendously from the scientific inquiry into postpartum depression. We know more today than ever about the phenomenon of PPD. But then, why is it still so prevalent? And if we know that most women who get PPD go undetected, what happens to them?

Moreover, what about women who score high on the screening instruments, those who meet diagnostic criteria (such that it is), who had risk factors that increase the likelihood of developing PPD, those who experienced the symptoms described in medical journals, those who undergo treatment that has been demonstrated to show some relief? What of them? Is that all there is? A laundry list of labels and recovery, and then it's over?

I knew from my own experience that the remnants of untreated PPD linger. Living through untreated PPD extends oneself beyond a previous point of identity; it marks a point on the map of one's life when things change forever. That is where I set up basecamp for this book.

In this new edition, I have included five new participants: Grace, Margery, Deborah, Adrienne, and Callie. While they responded to recruitment regarding postpartum depression, it became clear that the nature of their experiences mirrored those of the previous participants, but within a broader context of current reproductive technology, awareness of traumatic childbirth, and increased knowledge of the range of psychiatric disorders in the perinatal period. Their stories, combined with the original 20 participants and the survey research gathered from over 300 women, illustrate a definite conclusion. Untreated postpartum mood and anxiety disorders are the problems. The significance of the level of transformation noted in their stories is relative to the glaring fact that their disorders were not prevented. Their illness was generated by a system that failed them, not a body or a brain that was disordered.

Participants

I want to extend my gratitude to the 25 women who participated in interviews with me describing the experience of perinatal mood or anxiety disorders, postpartum psychosis, and traumatic birth identified by them as postpartum depression (PPD). Their experiences provide vital information regarding the power of PPD to decimate a woman's wellbeing and the potential of the human spirit to grow in spite of the destruction these disorders leave in their path.

Note: Pseudonyms have been used for all participants, and any identifying facts or details of their lives have been omitted to protect confidentiality. Participants have been listed in alphabetical order.

Anna, a 37-year-old professional fundraiser, and now stay-at-home mother described her journey as a reflection on a specific change in her appearance.

> When I was talking to my husband about this interview and that I was going to talk to you, he said, "You have to tell her about the earrings." When I graduated from high school, my grandparents gave me this beautiful pair of pearl earrings, and I wore them every day, and by saying I wore them every day, I literally mean those were the only pair of earrings I ever wore. Being a high school senior through [to] when my son was born. I wore those pearl earrings every day. I just considered it part of my identity. They were kind of a signature item. But now, I wear different jewelry all the time.

Beatrice, a 43-year-old psychologist, and prenatal yoga instructor also experienced PPD with both of her children, approximately six years before the time of the interview.

> First of all, it was long, I would say. It wasn't something that happened very quickly--I wouldn't call it an extended postpartum depression, but it certainly wasn't short.

Betsy, 35, an actress, author, and mother of two, began her long journey with PPD early after her birth.

> You know while I was in it, obviously it was all negative, but I think in the long term, I actually see it as what made my transformation into a mother complete because what I learned was so early on that there's no way to be perfect. There was going to be a lot that wasn't in my control and a lot that I didn't understand.

So, you know the time has given me the luxury of being able to see it that way.

Callie, a 42-year-old mother of two children, now ages 8 and 10. Callie had PPD with her second child and is currently working in the healthcare insurance industry. Callie divorced her husband after PPD, but they have since reunited. A critical aspect of Callie's experience of PPD was her choice to have an unmedicated childbirth with her second child. Callie's experience began, as she noted, "right at nine centimeters."

During the childbirth, when I was nine centimeters, and there was no going back, and I had no drugs, no epidural . . . I just remember hitting this place, when and it's, like, terrifying. Like, really having this moment of, "I can't go on, and this is all on my shoulders. And if I don't go on, I'm going to die, and my child is going to die." Just this perplexing-crashing-down-on-me emotional place. Because at that moment, I just put the brakes on. I was totally resistant to wanting any of this to happen anymore. That was an energy that carried through that I had to learn to cope with through the postpartum. Dana, a 40-year-old mother of three and an adjunct university instructor and public-health graduate student, experienced PPD following the birth of her second and third children, approximately six years before the interview.

After I wrote my book and released it, I realized my transformation. It was kind of like that's how I made peace with it, and I moved on.

Deborah, a 39-year-old elementary school teacher, and mother of a 6.5-year-old boy and 18-month-old daughter, experienced debilitating postpartum depression and anxiety following the birth of her son. She had been an active infertility blogger, sharing her struggle with Polycystic Ovarian Syndrome (PCOS) and infertility to get pregnant. For Deborah, anxiety manifested quickly and was exacerbated by lactation difficulties related to her PCOS.

Once my son came, it was pretty instant, I would say. At least within the first couple weeks that I started getting really overwhelming anxiety. He was a very difficult infant and a really difficult newborn. He had reflux, he cried constantly, and he cried through feedings. A big part of the start of all of this for me was that I had really bought into the "nursing is everything, and you have to nurse your baby, and nursing is what mothers do, and if you don't nurse, then you're . . ." Like, that overwhelming sort of breast is best stuff. But because of my polycystic ovary syndrome (PCOS), I physiologically could not nurse. I never lactated; I never got milk. I didn't know that then. Not being able to breastfeed was a huge anxiety trigger for me because he wasn't gaining weight, and he was screaming all the time, and I had 50 people telling me I was doing everything wrong. It just became incredibly overwhelming. That anxiety set in in the first couple weeks and then did not let up.

Diana, a 38-year-old full-time student, experienced PPD approximately two years before our interview, following the birth of both of her children, who were born only 11 months apart.

It was a slow progression getting better over time. I tried taking control of little things. I controlled what I could, but I still was completely out of control. And I tried, and I tried, and I tried. I tried "fake it until you make it" as long as I could. I definitely came out of it in baby steps.

Faith, a 48-year-old volunteer and mother of three experienced PPD following each of her births, more than 13 years ago.

My first postpartum depression lasted with the anxiety, approximately 15 months. I was very young; I was 22 when I gave birth to my first son. My second son was born when I was 26, and we were in a place physically, and financially, that was better than when we were so young with our first son. Then we waited nine years before, after the birth of the middle son, to have my third son. I think what blew me away about that experience is I thought I had it under control. My support system fell through, which began with my OB. It was quite scary. It took me 13 years to sign up to be able to volunteer to lead a postpartum support group. It took me that long to be able to be in a place in my head and with my educating myself with resources to feel confident to be able to help other women.

Georgia, a 42-year-old former documentary producer and current psychotherapist (licensed clinical social worker), has two children and experienced PPD following the birth of her first child. Georgia, when describing her sense of the speed of the transformation process, stated, *"Overall, the trajectory was, like, kind of slow and subtle."*

Grace, a 34-year-old woman, is the mother of two, postpartum doula and peer group facilitator, who experienced postpartum depression following the birth of her first child six years before the interview. Grace experienced PPD following an unexpected Cesarean section due to her baby being breech.

I think that's where it started. I, actually, looking back now know that I was depressed during my pregnancy because even though I had, like, a great pregnancy, he was breech at the end. And so, going from thinking I was going to have a typical birth and then finding out I was going to have to have a planned c-section was really devastating for me. We knew when he was coming, but I was really not happy about it. And then I had some provider experiences that were not great. Physically, everything went fine, but, you know, I was not doing well. I had symptoms pretty locked away, and you know, nobody was asking me, but it was like I had felt like I was in this tunnel vision in the last month of my pregnancy. Like, just making it to that day that he was going to be born. That day, I couldn't sleep and felt like this can't be happening--just a little bit disconnected from what was actually going on.

Haley, age 35, a full-time financial analyst, experienced PPD following the birth of her second child, 18 months before the interview.

I would say it took a while for me to kind of feel like myself again. I would say, at least a year.

Helena, a 43-year-old therapist who experienced PPD following the births of both of her daughters 12 years prior to our interview.

It was like a slow earthquake that, that had big shocks, and smaller shocks, but it was undermining the structural integrity of my identity as a person at the time until I could kind of regroup and build a different foundation.

Jamie, a 31-year-old high-level software tester in the technical industry, experienced PPD following the birth of her son, only two years before the interview.

One thing that's been extremely transformational was a year after he was born when my son's birthday came around, I went back to my therapist. One of the things I said was, "You know I just hated that hospital because all these people were touching me without my permission, and it just felt so awful." And she said, "Well, has that ever happened to you before? Has anybody done that to you before?" I was raped 14 years ago, and I never told anybody, and right then, I told her.

Janis, a 32-year-old master's level social-service professional, experienced PPD after the birth of her daughter, 10 months before the interview.

> *I think it took me a while that awareness of the parts of me that were transforming. I think for a while, I really—I externalized it. For a while and especially the first couple of months, I felt like it was something happening to me. So, it took a while to shift.*

Karen, a 30-year-old public health professional in a state agency, had experienced PPD two years before the interview.

> *Well, it was really slow., I mean, I guess in the long run, it feels fast, I guess right because it was only 2 years ago that it happened. But it's definitely felt slow during the process, right? I was diagnosed at around six weeks of postpartum. I'm almost two years out. So, I say that my transformation is still happening. I say that the initial transformation was just me coming to the realization that I could ask for help, that that was an okay thing.*

Margery, 34, is a married mother of two girls, ages 6 and 4. Margery experienced postpartum psychosis following the birth of her second child. Before her experience, she worked as a home health nurse. Margery's story sheds critical light on the dynamic of postpartum psychosis as mirroring that of women who had PPD. Since then, Margery quit full-time work and has dedicated herself to advocacy work for perinatal mood and anxiety disorder awareness.

> *You can't go through an experience like postpartum psychosis, and not come out on the other side with either some kind of diagnosis, whether it's generalized anxiety, like me, or bipolar, or something, and not want to make a change, and not be passionate about the future for yourself or other moms or your own children.*

But absolutely. I mean, I'm definitely not the same mom. I'm not the same person.

Mindy, a 45-year-old architectural lighting professional, experienced PPD following the birth of her second child, nearly three years before the interview. Her completion of a photography project about PPD almost a year after her experience.

It wasn't until I did my photography project where I was able to I think fully positively transform in my life and move forward because I realized at that point I didn't have to be stuck in these feelings, that that was part of my life, part of my pregnancy, part of my childbirth experience, but it didn't have to define me as a person.

Morgan, a 48-year-old financial industry professional, had experienced PPD following the birth of her daughter nearly seven years before the interview.

It wasn't until I was totally out of the fog that I realized, "Wow, I just experienced postpartum depression.

Paula, a 37-year-old quality professional, and mental-health blogger, shared that a particularly difficult moment leads to her realization of transformation sometime later,

I did have a really rough couple of weeks there just because in one of my more frustrated moments, I had told my husband that, "You need to take her because I'm afraid I might hurt her." I was just frustrated. She wouldn't nurse, she wouldn't settle down, and at that point, my husband didn't tell me until this incident happened several months ago, he said, "When you said that, I started making plans to what I would do if something happened."

Hearing that made me realize I was really, really struggling. But I'm better, and I can use my experience and my voice to help other moms realize they're not alone and it's okay to talk about these scary things because the more we talk about them, the more people can be educated and hopefully, we can prevent tragedies before they happen.

Sandy, a 32-year-old social media professional, experienced PPD following the birth of her first and second child.

Once you become depressed, you have to fight back to not only who you are, but you kind of have to let go of who you are and figure out who you are. And that in and of itself is very transformational because you're letting go of who you used to be because you're no longer that person. You're now a mother, and you have this child, and you're now battling a mental illness, which you may or may not have experience before giving birth.

You've got that, and then you're trying to figure what all of this makes you all at the same time. So yeah, I think overall, it's an extremely transformational process. I don't think I've talked to a single person ever who doesn't see it as such.

Sienna, a 28-year-old marketing communications specialist and mother of one, had experienced PPD five months before our interview.

My process of transformation through postpartum depression, it's been a very long road, but I think in the end, it has been transformational.

Skye, a 39-year-old professional counselor who experienced PPD with both children.

I didn't really come back very quickly. It took a really long time. And it really colored how I felt about myself.

Stephanie, a 29-year-old paralegal, experienced PPD following the birth of her first child, approximately one year before the interview.

I have come a long way since the darkness of that time.

Vicki, a 41-year-old advocate for a childhood tumor foundation, experienced PPD following the birth of her son, only a year before our interview.

It was a long journey of getting better. But it was definitely hard.

For the Reader

The stories shared by the 25 women in this book tell us what we need to know, what we must know about perinatal mood and anxiety disorders; that, left ignored, undetected, undiagnosed, and untreated, PPD deconstructed lives. Being unprepared for the symptoms begins a long journey of isolation, fear, terrifying confusion, and life-threatening thoughts.

Reading these experiences can be difficult. I considered trying to temper the material somehow. But there is no way to understand the breadth of the experience with watered-down language or paraphrase. Moreover, these are not my words; they are the words of women who know this experience first-hand, however they say it. Whatever language they use, we should listen closely. We should lean in to hear the differences, the silences, the repetitions and revelations of truth about postpartum depression.

CHAPTER 1

DEFINING POSTPARTUM DEPRESSION

*Some of the most powerful images of women and
motherhood are those held by the professional
disciplines which lay claim to a special expertise in
the field of reproduction—namely, medical science,
clinical psychiatry, and psychology.*
– Ann Oakley –

T he images of postpartum depression, as described by the
professions that have studied it, create a collage of definitions,
diagnoses, treatments, measurements, and theories considered
by medical science, nursing, psychology, psychiatry, and to a
lesser extent, a small number of feminist theories from sociology.
This chapter provides an overview of the research regarding PPD,
as defined by the professionals who have studied it. Part I reviews
current clinical definitions and prevalence rates for postpartum
depression; Part II surveys the literature regarding risk factors,
and Part III presents substantive literature regarding the effects
of PPD on women and children.

PART I:
WHAT IS POSTPARTUM DEPRESSION?

Globally, health institutions grapple with the language of PPD.
The World Health Organization (WHO) defines PPD as "a clinical and research construct used to describe an episode of major

or minor depression arising after childbirth" (WHO, 2009, p. 17). According to the *Diagnostic and Statistical Manual, 5th Edition* postpartum depression refers to a "nonpsychotic depressive episode that begins in the postpartum period" (American Psychiatric Association [APA], 2013, p. 160). The word postpartum in both cases is used as an onset specifier for a diagnosis of Major Depressive Disorder (MDD). In other words, from a medical standpoint, PPD is a major depression that happens after childbirth.

PPD symptoms are consistent with those in MDD (Preston & Johnson, 2009), with one huge exception: motherhood. Women who have PPD are experiencing a full-blown episode of major depression in addition to the increased demands of caring for a newborn and recovering from childbirth. Leading PPD researcher Michael O'Hara (2009) noted:

> *Major depression creates suffering, whether experienced in the postpartum period or at any other time in a woman's life. What makes depression so poignant for postpartum women is that childbirth is culturally celebrated, and there is an expectation that new parents, especially mothers, will be joyful, if not tired, during this time. Moreover, the demands on a new mother are substantial and include providing 24-hour care for a newborn, often in the middle of the night, caring for older children, keeping up with normal household responsibilities, and often returning to work after brief maternity leave. These burdens are often difficult to bear in normal circumstances, and the difficulty of bearing them is exacerbated by the disability associated with depression symptoms* (p. 1259).

O'Hara's (2009) description resonates; PPD *is* different. It is an experience of psychiatric illness during a life event unlike any other: motherhood. However, in the eyes of medical science, PPD is still defined as an MDD that sometimes can occur in women after childbirth.

Since the first use of postpartum specifiers in the *Diagnostic and Statistical Manual, 3rd Edition (DSM-3)* (APA, 1994), the timing was set at four weeks following the birth of a baby. Clinical experts have petitioned for expanding that timeframe based on what they are seeing in their patients, that symptoms of PPD can arise three to six months after childbirth. The most recent *DSM-5* (APA, 2013) extended the timing to six weeks postpartum, the same timing noted in the *International Classification of Diseases-10* (ICD-10-CM; WHO, 2015).

Defining PPD: The Diagnostic Manuals

In essence, the diagnostic manuals that describe physical and psychiatric illnesses do not have specific diagnostic criteria for PPD or other perinatal mood and anxiety disorders such as postpartum anxiety, bipolar disorder, posttraumatic stress disorder, or psychosis. There is no separate and equal category of reproductive psychiatric disorders in medical diagnostic manuals. In effect, women's reproductive psychiatric illnesses remain in the shadow of the dominant paradigm of disease classification.

How this translates for women and providers is important. When women have symptoms, there is no clear description for the care provider to consult, a medical code to chart, or treatment protocol associated with the disorder recognized by health insurance.

Unpacking this a bit further, we can understand that the lack of a specific clinical diagnostic classification for PPD reveals a tepid understanding of the phenomenon itself, by people who made the manual. This lack of diagnostic legitimacy in the current dominant medical paradigm creates a tacit, yet powerful (if not intentional) disconnect between women's reproduction psychology. Are we in ancient, silent agreement with Hippocrates—that the womb of a woman had a mind of its own, wandering around irrationally, creating inherent and gendered psychological imbalance?

What Postpartum Depression is Not

A dangerous mixture of stigma and media has led to an accepted association between the word *postpartum* and the most tragic of cases involving infanticide. Confusion in media reporting fuels devastating stereotypes that marginalize mothers and creates powerful social obstacles to seeking help.

Media reports misinterpreting the research regarding the safety of psychiatric medication during pregnancy and postpartum can have dangerous implications for women who choose to discontinue medication without a proper medical assessment. There is a significant absence of media reports regarding trauma in pregnancy and postpartum women, both in our military servicewomen and the civilian population. There is an overwhelming sensationalist portrayal of our most tragic cases of perinatal psychosis that leads to infanticide, and relatively little reporting on the instances of perinatal suicide, self-harm, negative impact on children, or the new understanding of the role of bipolar.

What we do know is that there is a spectrum of psychological diagnoses during the perinatal period, ranging from the mildest, postpartum blues, to the most severe, postpartum psychosis (O'Hara & Segre, 2008).

Postpartum Blues

Postpartum blues is described as "mood lability, irritability, interpersonal hypersensitivity, insomnia, anxiety, tearfulness, and sometimes elation" (O'Hara, 2009, p. 1259). Postpartum blues, maternity blues, or "baby blues" (Bennett & Indman, 2019, p. 34) was introduced to the medical literature by Maloney (1952) as "third-day depression" (p. 21). Postpartum blues presents mild, time-limited symptoms of depression, such as irritability, mood swings, and tearfulness occurring soon after childbirth and resolving within 10 to 14 days following childbirth (O'Hara & Segre, 2008). Postpartum blues are reported to occur from 50% to 80% of mothers following childbirth (O'Hara & Wisner, 2014). Usually, postpartum blues resolves itself without treatment but remains a risk factor for the more severe PPD (O'Hara & Wisner, 2014; O'Keane et al., 2011).

Perinatal Anxiety Disorders

Given the comorbidity of depression and anxiety symptoms, research on perinatal anxiety disorders is still evolving (Agius et al., 2016; Dikmen-Yildiz et al., 2017). Perinatal anxiety, OCD, panic disorder, and phobias have been noted in the literature and continue to receive more scientific focus (Fawcett et al., 2019; Miller et al., 2015a, 2015b; Reck et al., 2008).

Bipolar Disorder

Childbirth is an established risk factor for the onset or recurrence of a BD in the postpartum period (Sharma et al., 2014). The post-partum period represents the highest lifetime risk for both first-time onset and recurrence for bipolar disorder (Wisner et al., 2013). High prevalence of bipolar disorders in the postpartum period: 0-12 months following childbirth (Wisner et al., 2013). One US study has reported prevalence for BD in past-year pregnant women at 2-8% (Vesga-Lopez et al., 2008).

A nationally representative study of an obstetric sample of 10,000 women found that 22.6% screened positive for bipolar disorders (Wisner et al., 2013). Stigma remains a powerful barrier to women seeking help for symptoms of bipolar disorder in the perinatal period (Ladd, 2018).

Postpartum Psychosis

As noted, at the other end of the spectrum of perinatal mental illness is the most severe and life-threatening disorder: postpartum psychosis. Postpartum psychosis affects one to two women per 1,000 births globally, and while rare, it is an extremely severe postpartum mood disorder and is a psychiatric emergency that requires immediate medical attention (O'Hara & Wisner, 2014).

The description of the spectrum of perinatal mood and anxiety disorders sheds further light on how the professions charged with reproduction have identified symptoms and modeled diagnoses. Psychiatry, driven by empirical science, have been charged with measuring the rates postpartum mood and anxiety disorders in our population. Note the absence of the word trauma or the inclusion of traumatic stress symptoms in these disorders

How Common is Postpartum Depression?

Within the spectrum of postpartum blues and postpartum psychosis, postpartum depression occurs in approximately 1 in 7 women, with current literature suggesting an overall prevalence range of 10-18% for the occurrence of PPD in the general population (Curry et al., 2019; Fisher et al., 2012; Gavin et al., 2005; Patel et al., 2012).

What is Prevalence?

Prevalence is an estimated measurement of how common a condition occurs in the population, or "a proportion of people affected by a specific characteristic during a specific time" (NIMH, 2017). Prevalence is calculated by taking a random sample of people with the characteristic in a small sample divided by the total number of people in the sample:

Since writing the first edition, some critical developments have emerged regarding the prevalence of PPD globally. Namely, there is a much broader range of prevalence rates than previously reported, and secondly, that the prevalence is still high. A 2019 literature review of 203 studies conducted between 2005 and 2014 suggested that "The current prevalence of PPD is much higher than that previously reported" (Slomian et al., 2019, p. 34). However, there is a wide range of prevalence rates within the body of research examining PPD in developed versus developing countries and based on race and socioeconomic status.

Global Prevalence

Data on global rates of PPD demonstrate substantial evidence that PPD is not culturally bound (Eberhard-Gran et al., 2010; Prabhu et al., 2019). In an early landmark study, Kumar (1994) presented robust findings that "there are no major differences in rates of postnatal depression in the few cross-cultural comparisons that have so far been reported" (p. 256). The WHO (2001) reported that for all women aged 15 to 44 years, major depression, not only PPD, but all types of depression, is second only to HIV/AIDS in terms of total disability. The Global Burden of Disease for women who have a mental illness is profound.

The range of reported prevalence rates internationally is between 1.9% and 82.1% in developed countries, with the lowest prevalence reported in Germany (Halbreich & Karkun, 2006).

A 2019 national retrospective cohort study of 381,685 United Kingdom mothers tracked through the Clinical Practice Research Datalink (CPRD) between 2005 and 2017 determined an overall prevalence of maternal mental illness at 23.2% with depression and anxiety as the most common disorders. The authors concluded that based on their data, "One in four children aged 0–16 years are exposed to maternal mental illness and the prevalence of diagnosed and treated maternal mental illness is increasing" (Abel et al., 2019, p. e291). While the prevalence rates may not reflect the presence of just PPD, the study demonstrates the range of research findings on the global prevalence of maternal mental illness.

Developing Countries

Studies have demonstrated a variance in prevalence rates in developing countries as well (Bener et al., 2012; Slomian et al., 2019), citing Pakistan as having the lowest prevalence rate of 5.2% and Turkey having the highest at 74.0% (Norhayati et al., 2015). Conversely, a systematic review of 1,000 prevalence studies reported an overall rate of 19.8%, a much higher prevalence than high-income countries (Fisher et al., 2012).

Onset and Prevalence

While the majority of research has agreed on the timing of symptoms, more recent research has suggested a higher prevalence in the prenatal period. A 2017 study of a representative sample of 3,233 mothers in the Czech Republic noted higher prevalence before delivery (12.8%) than at 6 weeks postpartum (11.89%) and at 6 months postpartum (10.1%) suggesting prenatal prevalence for mood and anxiety disorder is higher than previously reported (Fiala et al., 2017).

It has been suggested that the reason for the uncertainty in prevalence rate reports is the differences in screening protocol or absence of screening protocol: "Depending on the definition of the disorder, country, diagnostic tools used, threshold of discrimination chosen for the screening measure, and period over which prevalence is determined" (Slomian et al., 2019, p. 2). The numbers, while ranging widely, still signify an alarmingly high presence of PPD in birthing women and adoptive moms and dads. Epidemiological data suggest that race and socioeconomic factors contribute to a higher prevalence among communities of color.

Prevalence Rates and Race

PPD has been shown to affect rural, low-income women of color disproportionately (Collado et al., 2014; Jesse & Swanson, 2007; Knitzer et al., 2008; Melville et al., 2010; Segre et al., 2007). Studies demonstrate that approximately 30-40% of Latina women living in the United States experience perinatal mood and anxiety disorders, three times that of the general U. S. population (Chaudron et al., 2005; Lucero et al., 2012), yet may be less likely to report being depressed (Chaudron, 2005; Segre et al., 2006).

Prevalence rates among African American, Hispanic, and Native American women have been reported as disproportionately high compared to white women, yet the rates vary widely in overall reporting. The influence of racial/ethnic disparities in care on the reporting of depressive symptoms has yet to be thoroughly examined (Liu & Tronick, 2014; Mukherjee et al., 2016). Factors of discrimination, violence, poverty, and stigma regarding mental health have been reported as contributors to women of color not seeking mental healthcare (Chaudron, 2005; Nadeem et al., 2007).

A 2010 nationally representative study of (N = 3,051) pregnant women determined that "non-white and Hispanic women without a history of mental health were less likely to report poor antepartum mental health" (Witt et al., 2010, p. 433). Other studies have suggested that ethnic underrepresentation in mental health research, less satisfaction with services received, or negative beliefs about treatment contribute to underestimating prevalence for minority women in the United States (McGuire et al., 2006; Stockman et al., 2015; Wang et al., 2005).

Prevalence rates among African American, Hispanic, and Native American women may be underestimated (Taylor & Kuo, 2019). The influence of racial/ethnic disparities in care on the reporting of depressive symptoms has yet to be thoroughly examined (Breslau et al., 2005). Factors of discrimination, violence, poverty, stigma regarding mental health, preferential diagnosis among Caucasian women, compared to minority women, have been reported as contributors to women of color not seeking mental healthcare (Nadeem et al., 2007).

A 2010 nationally representative study of (N = 3,051) pregnant women determined that "non-white and Hispanic women without a history of mental health were less likely to report poor ante-partum mental health" (Witt et al., 2010, p. 433). Other studies have suggested that ethnic underrepresentation in mental health research, less satisfaction with services received, or negative beliefs about treatment contribute to underestimating preva-lence for minority women in the United States (McGuire et al., 2006). Segre et al. (2006) examined race/ethnicity as a risk factor for depressed mood in late pregnancy and the early postpartum period, reporting that African American women were signifi-cantly more likely to report depressed mood, while Hispanic American women were significantly less likely to report being depressed.

Research shows that U.S. Hispanic mothers may be less likely to use mental health care services as compared to other minority women, regardless of income or insurance coverage (Shellman et al., 2014). Systemic barriers to treatment for Latinas may be so pervasive as to skew the prevalence rates altogether (Abrams et al., 2009; Kozhimannil et al., 2011). In a study of (N = 218) Hispanic new mothers, Chaudron et al. (2005) reported 28% of mothers self-identified as needing help with depression since the birth of their baby, and less than half had discussed depression with a care provider. A 2011 retrospective cohort study of childbearing women enrolled in New Jersey's Medicaid program reported that that African American and Latina mothers were significantly less likely to seek help for postpartum depression than Caucasian mothers (Kozhimannil et al., 2011).

The takeaway regarding prevalence might be that while the research notes a wide range within categories of developed and developing countries, the rates remain high universally, and consistently higher for women living in poverty, and women of color in the United States (Canady et al., 2008). PPD affects women globally and pervasively.

Knowing something is wrong and yet not sharing it with a care provider is part of the picture of PPD that we have yet to study or understand fully. Notably, the literature examines why women are less likely to engage in what is called "help-seeking behavior" versus why healthcare providers fail to screen and treat women. As we see in the stories of the women presented in this book, even when women told multiple providers they were ill, the providers failed to meet the help-seeking behavior with help-giving behavior, such as screening women for risk factors known to increase a woman's chance of experiencing PPD.

PART II: RISK FACTORS

An explanation of the risk factors experienced before and during pregnancy leads to a better understanding of the physical, psychological, and socioeconomic conditions associated with the probability of developing PPD. Goodman and Dimidjian (2012) define risk in this way:

> *Risk is defined as a condition that increases the probability of developing a disorder. A risk factor necessarily precedes the onset of the disorder and is difficult to identify empirically, as prospective longitudinal designs are required. More research has focused on correlates of depression (that is, factors that tend to co-occur with depression rather than risk)* (p. 532).

What follows is a brief description of the current literature regarding what we know regarding the increased risk of developing PPD in the areas of (a) maternal history of a mood or anxiety disorder, (b) reproductive and obstetric risk factors, and (c) psychosocial risk factors. I also reference new research interests regarding genetic and epigenetic risk factors.

History of Mood or Anxiety Disorder

Prior history of mental health problems has been shown as a significant risk factor for the development of PPD (Howard et al., 2018; Lancaster et al., 2010; Mora et al., 2009; Munk-Olsen et al., 2019).

Depression during pregnancy has also been reported as a significant risk factor for the development of PPD (Goodman & Tully, 2009; Howard et al., 2014; Howard et al., 2018; Leigh & Milgrom, 2008; Munk-Olsen et al., 2019). In a frequently cited systematic review, Gaynes et al. (2005) reported that 14.5% of women developed a new episode of major or minor depression in pregnancy.

Mental health problems are common during pregnancy, with as many as one-in-four women meeting diagnostic criteria for a mental disorder in early pregnancy, with anxiety disorders and depression being the most common conditions (Howard et al., 2018; Munk-Olsen et al., 2019). As well as the morbidity experienced by the mother, maternal mental disorders may be associated with obstetric complications (Accortt et al., 2015) and developmental difficulties in the offspring (Stein et al., 2014). A woman's reproductive health and wellbeing are not separate from her mental health and wellbeing. Reproduction itself creates many of the conditions for the onset of perinatal mood and anxiety disorders.

Reproductive or Obstetric Risk Factors

While the majority of extant literature reports that first-time mothers, older mothers, and young mothers have a higher risk of developing PPD (Munk-Olsen et al., 2019; Records & Rice, 2007; U.S. CDC, 2008; Vesga-Lopez et al., 2008), more recent literature notes that recurrence patterns in multiparous women demonstrate significantly higher risk (Munk-Olsen et al., 2019).

Unplanned or Unwanted Pregnancy

Unplanned or unwanted pregnancy has also been demonstrated as a risk factor for PPD (Fisher et al., 2012; Lancaster et al., 2010; Lee, et al., 2007; Mora et al., 2009; Rich-Edwards et al., 2006). Women with a history of obstetric complications, such as stillbirth or miscarriage, may be at increased risk of developing PPD (Abebe, et al., 2019; Azad et al., 2019).

Mode of Delivery

There are mixed findings regarding an increased risk of PPD and mode of delivery (Declerq et al., 2013; Gaillard et al., 2014). Some recent research has reported no increased risk for women experiencing PPD based on mode of delivery (Bell et al., 2018), while other studies have indicated a correlation between unplanned cesarean sections and increased risk of PPD (Koutra, et al., 2018; Sarah et al., 2017).

Postpartum Hemorrhage

Additionally, the experience of postpartum hemorrhage, and preeclampsia may be associated with increased risk of PPD (Borra et al., 2015; Eckerdal et al., 2016; Figueiredo et al., 2013; Hamdan & Tamim, 2012; Koutra et al., 2018).

Psychosocial Risk Factors

Research has reported that women with low self-esteem are at higher risk for PPD (Jesse & Swanson, 2007; Leigh & Milgrom, 2008; Sharifzadeh et al., 2018; Zaidi et al., 2018). Also, women with perceived lack of social support are at higher risk for experiencing PPD (Gan et al., 2019; Lancaster et al., 2010; Leigh & Milgrom, 2008; Vaezi et al., 2019; Westdahl et al., 2007).

Non-partnered or unmarried mothers are at increased risk for developing PPD, as are mothers in unhappy partnerships, or marriages (Lancaster et al., 2010; Records & Rice, 2007; Wszołek et al., 2018). In a systematic review, Fisher et al. (2012) reported that for pregnant and postpartum women in low- and lower-to-middle-income countries, psychosocial risk factors included (a) being unmarried; (b) lack of intimate partner support; (c) having hostile in-laws; (d) lack of emotional or practical support; and (e) intimate partner violence.

Socioeconomic and Cultural Risk Factors

Poverty has been associated with increased life stress and depression in the general population since the latter part of the 20th century (Holmes & Rahe, 1967). It is not surprising, therefore, that poor women are at higher risk of experiencing PPD as reported extensively in the literature (Kosidou et al., 2011; Lancaster et al., 2010; Leigh & Milgrom, 2008; Munk-Olsen et al., 2019; Priest, et al., 2008; Sahrakorpi et al., 2017).

In a study with a large sample of postpartum women (N= 4,332), Segre et al. (2007) reported income as a reliable predictor for PPD, and that low occupational prestige, marital status, and numbers of children were also significant predictors.

The Combination of Risk Factors

The research regarding risk factors has demonstrated that PPD does not occur in isolation, but rather, in "conjunction with a complex interplay of sociodemographic, biophysical, psychosocial, and behavioral factors" (Jesse & Swanson, 2007, p. 378). The previous history of mental health problems, maternal age, obstetric problems, unplanned pregnancies, lack of social support, violence in the home, and poverty have all been found as correlates to the development of PPD (Guintivano et al., 2018). The pathways through which these factors create risk have been of interest to the field of epigenetics.

Genetic and Epigenetic Factors

There has been an increased interest in understanding genetic connections to PPD in the last decade. Several studies have reported a positive relationship between the serotonin transporter gene 5HTTLRP and the development of PPD (Binder et al., 2010; eCouto et al., 2015). A more recent matched prospective observational study demonstrated lipidomic biomarkers associated with depression for women who had a cesarean birth (Wu et al., 2019).

PART III: WHAT ARE THE EFFECTS OF PPD?

The research regarding the effects of PPD on mothers and their infants has been substantial. I first offer a brief overview of the research on the effects of PPD on women. Secondly, I review some of the effects of PPD on infants and children.

Maternal Mortality

Major depression is a risk for suicide. As we have learned in this chapter, PPD is defined as an episode of major depression after having a baby. Therefore, it is not surprising that suicide is one of the leading causes of maternal mortality during the first year after childbirth (Bodnar-Deren et al., 2016; Howard et al., 2011; Lewis, 2007; Oyston et al., 2017; Palladino et al., 2011; Paris et al., 2009; Shi et al., 2018).

An early study from the United Kingdom, Oates (2003) reported that of the total 378 incidences of maternal death (death within 42 days postpartum), between the years 1997 and 1999, suicide was the leading cause of death. More recently, Knight (2019) reported suicide as the third leading cause of death in the UK, according to the MBRRACE-UK confidential inquiry into Maternal Deaths and Morbidity.

In the United States, a 2005 review reported suicides accounting for 20% of deaths; and the percentage of mothers with thoughts of self-harm during pregnancy and postpartum ranged from 5% to 14% (Lindahl et al., 2005). More recently, researchers analyzed the death records for women of reproductive age who died between 2003 and 2007, using the CDC's National Violent Death Reporting System (Palladino et al., 2011). The report stated that "the rates of pregnancy-associated homicide and suicide were each higher than mortality rates attributable to common obstetric causes" (Palladino et al., 2011, p. 1059). Moreover, 51% of the suicides occurred during the postpartum period. Victims were significantly more likely to be unmarried, and either Caucasian or Native American. In 54% of the cases, intimate partner conflict contributed to suicide (Palladino et al., 2011).

Suicidal Ideation

The precursor to all suicide in most cases is suicidal ideation, or intrusive thoughts of suicide, and the presence of major depression (Gavin et al., 2011; Gelabert et al., 2019; Mauri et al., 2012; Perez-Rodriguez, et al., 2008). Howard et al. (2011) examined suicidal ideation in a large (N = 4,150) sample of postpartum women using the Edinburgh Postnatal Depression Scale (EPDS) (Cox et al., 1987). Nine percent of 4,150 women reported some suicidal ideation, and 4% reported thoughts of harming themselves occurring sometimes or quite often.

Given that the majority of women who get PPD go untreated or undetected (Cox et al., 2016; Elisei et al., 2013; Ko et al., 2016), and the rates of completed suicides in the postpartum period remains relatively low, it is safe to argue that we have little idea as to how frequently women experience suicidal ideation postpartum. For the mothers in my study, there was a shocking relationship between suicide and PPD that must be explored in future research.

What does it do to a woman to be a mother of an infant and want to die? How is the experience of those thoughts while caring for a newborn resolved, recovered, or remembered? A 2016 nationally representative study of suicidal ideation and behavior among pregnant women in the United States showed that while the rates of suicidal behavior remained unchanged, the rates of suicidal ideation in pregnant women doubled between the years 2006-2012 (Zhong et al., 2016). Suicidal ideation was higher among African American women and women at or below the poverty line. Young women, ages 12-18, had the highest rate of suicidal behavior per pregnancy. While most suicidal behaviors were associated with depression, "more than 30% of hospitalizations were for suicidal behavior without depression diagnoses" (Zhong et al., 2016, p. 463).

Similar findings were reported in a 2017 study of suicidal ideation and behavior (SIB) among 376 pregnant women. While depression and anxiety disorders were associated with SIB, 67% did not have a diagnosis of depression, 65% had no diagnosis of anxiety, and 54% had neither a diagnosis of depression nor anxiety (Onah et al., 2017). The authors noted that socioeconomic factors, food insecurity, previous suicide attempts, and interpersonal violence were contributing factors that warrant providers screening for suicide risk "independently of depression and anxiety" (Onah et al., 2017, p. 321). Hall et al. (2019) also demonstrated a relationship between the previous history of self-harm and increased risk of mood and anxiety disorders in an early pregnancy sample of 544 women.

A 2018 study of maternal depression and suicide among 213 Chinese women, suicidal ideation was reported more frequently after childbirth (11.74%) than before birth (5.16 %) but scored lower on depression scales in the postpartum period (Shi et al., 2018). Lower depression but higher suicidal ideation during early postpartum was a novel finding that suggests that the relationship between depression and suicidal ideation is a complex correlation that warrants more research.

Effects of Depression on the Mother's Physical Health

We know that depression has immediate and longer-term negative effects on women. Long-term physical effects of major depression in the general population have been reported, suggesting that postpartum depression may put women at increased risk for developing future mental and physical problems (Abdollahi & Zargami, 2018; Slomian et al., 2019). Postpartum depression is also an established risk for recurrent depressive episodes along the lifespan (Letourneau et al., 2010). Depression is a known risk factor for heart disease in women (Pan et al., 2011; Schnatz et al., 2011). Depression has also been associated with an increased risk for stroke (O'Donnell et al., 2010), Alzheimer's disease, dementia, and cognitive impairment in later life (Rosenberg et al., 2010; Saczynski et al., 2010; Wilson et al., 2010; Wint, 2011).

Symptoms of mood and anxiety disorders can significantly impair a woman's ability to administer self-care, disrupting her ability to respond to her physical needs, and those of her infant (Barkin, & Wisner, 2013; Bernstein et al., 2008; Haga et al., 2012; Slomian et al., 2019). It is not uncommon for women to suffer from more than one mood or anxiety disorder at a time. When this happens, co-occurring mood and anxiety disorders often contribute to impairing maternal self-care and, in turn, a woman's ability to care for her infant (Henshaw, 2007; Murray et al., 2007; Paris et al., 2009; Slomian et al., 2019).

For example, eating disorders have been reported in the postpartum period (Kimmel et al., 2016; Riquin et al., 2019). When an eating disorder occurs at the same time as PPD, a woman and her baby are at higher risk of nutritional deficiency

(Nunes-Cortez, 2010). When more than one disorder occurs, such as obsessive-compulsive disorder (OCD), panic disorder, or posttraumatic stress disorder (PTSD) women experience even higher risks of impaired sleep, eating difficulties, lack of concentration, and thought regulation (Bowen et al., 2009). Substance abuse can co-occur with PPD, impairing a woman's ability to meet basic needs for herself or her infant, and increased risk of accident, risk-taking behavior, and suicide attempts (Bruce et al., 2008; McNamara et al., 2019; Ross & Dennis, 2009).

Effects of Maternal Depression on Children

We know that PPD has negative effects on infants, children, and adolescents (Campbell et al., 2007; Goodman & Tully, 2009; McNamara et al., 2019; Mora et al., 2009; Murray et al., 2011). Many studies have demonstrated that young children exposed to maternal depression exhibit more physical ailments (Chee, et al., 2008) and behavior problems (Campbell et al., 2009; Cents et al., 2013).

An association between maternal depression and insecure attachment to mothers in infancy has been well-established in the literature (Davis et al., 2019; McNamara et al., 2019; Murray et al., 2011). Exposure to maternal depression before the age of 2 has been associated with increased risk for depression in offspring up to and through adolescence (Davis et al., 2020; Halligan et al., 2007; Hay et al., 2008; Letourneau et al., 2013).

The severity and chronicity of a mother's symptoms influence the children's symptoms. The more severe and chronic the mother's symptoms, the more the symptoms the children are likely to have. The severity and chronicity of mothers' depression often co-occur with socioeconomic risk factors and racial/ethnic minority status (Pascoe et al., 2006). Postpartum depression has also been demonstrated to negatively impact the mother-child relationships over the lifespan (Myers & Johns, 2018). Severe and chronic maternal depression create the causes for more significant impact on children, underscoring the urgent importance for all health care providers to address the needs of women during the perinatal period. The research provides a distressing image of the deleterious effects of PPD, yet so many women remain untreated.

At the beginning of this chapter, I referenced Ann Oakley's (1993) statement regarding the images of women and motherhood as constructed by "the professional disciplines which lay claim to a special expertise in the field of reproduction—namely, medical science, clinical psychiatry, and psychology" (p. 19). An integral part of the constructs of PPD is based in a large part to the use of validated screening instruments that successfully and reliably report and predict the onset of PPD.

Cracks in the Image: Screening for PPD

Perinatal mood and anxiety disorders are not coincidental psychiatric events. The onset of disorders is related to the hormonal fluctuations of the endocrine system and subsequent shapeshifting of the brain during pregnancy and postpartum. Decades of perinatal psychiatric research demonstrate evidence that these disorders are part of the spectrum of effects of reproductive life events. Furthermore, screening instruments have been validated in the literature for nearly 30 years (Ukatu et al., 2018). These self-inventories include the Edinburgh Postnatal Depression Scale (EPDS; Cox et al., 1987); the CESD-R revised (Eaton et al., 2004); the Patient Health Questionnaire (PHQ-9; Spitzer et al., 1999); the Patient Health Questionnaire-2 (PHQ-2; Kroenke et al., 2003; and the Postpartum Depression Screening Scale (PPDS; Beck & Gable, 2000). Many of these self-inventories are available at no cost and online.

Consider for a moment that one scale, the PHQ-2 (Kroenke et al., 2003), is validated to accurately screen for depression using two questions within one stem question:

Over the past two weeks, how often have you been bothered by any of the following problems? 1) Little interest or pleasure in doing things; and 2) Feeling down, depressed, or hopeless

Now consider that the American College of Obstetricians and Gynecologists (ACOG) does not mandate that OB-GYN's screen for depression during pregnancy or postpartum. Granted, ACOG is a professional organization and cannot mandate what individual practitioners do but recommend a set of standards of practice. The recommendation, is as follows:

It is recommended that all obstetrician–gynecologists and other obstetric care providers complete a full assessment of mood and emotional well-being (including screening for postpartum depression and anxiety with a validated instrument) during the comprehensive postpartum visit for each patient. If a patient is screened for depression and anxiety during pregnancy, additional screening should then occur during the comprehensive postpartum visit. There is evidence that screening alone can have clinical benefits, although initiation of treatment or referral to mental health care providers offers maximum benefit. (ACOG, 2010)

Data are clear that screening works, yet, the obstetric opinions to screen for these disorders remain tepid at best.

It is not that ACOG is shy in educating women about routine tests to expect during pregnancy. For example, the patient information of routine tests during pregnancy currently on the ACOG website provides information regarding tests done in early pregnancy:

- Complete blood count (CBC)

- Blood type

- Urinalysis

- Urine culture

- Rubella

- Hepatitis B and hepatitis C

- Sexually transmitted infections (STIs)

- Human immunodeficiency virus (HIV)

- Tuberculosis (TB)

- The tests done in later pregnancy are noted:

- A repeat CBC

- Rh antibody test

- Glucose screening test

- Group B streptococci (GBS)

Yet, there is no test, nor terminology on the FAQ sheet related to screening for mental health during pregnancy, but there is a fact sheet on a different linked page.

In advertising its newly revised book *Pregnancy: Month by Month* ACOG (2010) lists common questions pregnant women ask their providers.

Whether you're thinking about getting pregnant or have already received the good news, this authoritative book provides you with useful advice from OB/GYNs:

- How do I know if I'm pregnant? What are the early signs and symptoms of pregnancy?

- Which prenatal genetic tests are best for my family and me?

- What can I expect during pregnancy checkups with my OB/GYN?

- What if I have morning sickness? How do I control morning sickness? When do nausea and vomiting most often occur during pregnancy?

- Can I exercise during pregnancy? When should I begin to exercise during pregnancy? What exercises are safe during pregnancy?

- What's a good pregnancy diet? Should my diet change month by month? Are there foods to avoid during pregnancy? Is it safe to eat sushi during pregnancy? How much caffeine is safe during pregnancy?

- Is it safe to color my hair during pregnancy?

- When will I hear my baby's heartbeat?

- What does fetal development look like month by month? When can an ultrasound tell my baby's sex?

- How do the placenta and umbilical cord form during pregnancy?

- What is preeclampsia? What are the signs and symptoms of preeclampsia?

- What about pain relief during labor?

- What are good exercises to do after pregnancy to help tone my "core?"

- What about breastfeeding or bottle feeding?

- Does bleeding during pregnancy mean I'm having a miscarriage?

Sometimes what is absent explains more than what is present. The total absence of mental health questions in this "authoritative" book on pregnancy and childbirth speaks to a dangerous gap in practice. ACOG has made recent attempts to advance its position on the need to screen postpartum patients, acknowledging that perinatal depression is "one of the most common medical complications during pregnancy and the postpartum period, affecting one in seven women" (ACOG, 2018, e208). Notably, nearly 50% of women are not screened (Elisei, 2013), and as many as 40% of women don't attend the postpartum visit (Bennet et al., 2014).

CONCLUSION

Since writing the first edition of this book, the prevalence rates, risk factors, and effects of PPD remain alarmingly persistent in the published literature. A well-studied cluster of completely preventable and treatable illnesses have not been prevented nor adequately treated, leaving women like the 25 profiled in the next chapters, unprepared for the onset of PPD and vulnerable to prolonged suffering.

CHAPTER 2

BEFORE POSTPARTUM DEPRESSION: I WAS UNPREPARED

Whether we like it or not, each of us, because
he has a human brain, forms a theory of reality that
brings order into what otherwise would be a chaotic
world experience. We need a theory to
make sense out of the world.

– Seymour Epstein–

In approaching a description of the first phase of transformation through untreated traumatic PPD, it is important to understand how women structure reality before PPD. The seminal work of psychologist Seymour Epstein sheds early light on psychology's understanding of the intricate web of assumptions about the world and self-identity in cognitive functioning. Epstein (1980) suggested that we form a central theory of reality made up of two distinctive sub-theories—a theory about ourselves and a theory about the world. Cognitive psychology supports the theory of theories, demonstrating that our brains process sensory information throughout our lives in ways that create paradigms, schemas, or assumptions of our world. These assumptions form a foundation of who we are and how we predict our world to treat us.

HOW WE SEE OUR WORLD

Throughout our lives, our cognitive functions of learning, problem-solving, memory, and language process sensory information, creating knowledge of ourselves, others, and our environment. Through cognition, systems of mental representations, called heuristics, we patch together assumptions about how things are in the world. We perceive the mental representations as solid constructs, and the patterns of activity between them as predictable behavior painting our reality. Learning these patterns, believing our assumptions of predictability, creates our concepts of who we are and how the world will treat us.

When new information is presented, we attribute most of it to our pre-existing assumptions, assigning the information to its designated mental construct and set of behaviors, memories, images, and emotions. We function on basic assumptions about our world created through the cognitive road mapping that begins at birth.

The work of Epstein and many others in cognitive and trauma psychology suggests that most of us share three assumptions (Janoff-Bulman & Frieze, 1983) that co-create our theory of reality: 1) the belief we are safe (invulnerability), 2) the belief that our world makes sense in meaningful ways (purpose and predictability), and 3) the belief that we are positive agents in our world. More recently, Janoff-Bulman (2011, p. 6) distilled these three assumptions into the idea that at some level, we all believe:

- The world is benevolent
- The world is meaningful
- The self is worthy

These beliefs provide a structure for how we sense and perceive our world. However, when events occur that change cognition at its core, our world is no longer benevolent, nor meaningful, and we experience profound psychological distress. Disruptive events can be organic such as diseases or illnesses affecting cognitive functioning, or traumatic such as traumatic brain injury or accidents. Mental illnesses can also reconfigure cognitive functioning, along with substance or alcohol abuse and addiction. Research regarding the witnessing of traumatic events, where one's life or the lives of others is at risk, or being the victim of the assault has demonstrated that exposure to traumatic life events also changes cognitive functioning, altering how we see the world and its predictability in light of altered hardwiring of the brain.

The experience of untreated PPD shattered assumptions about the world as benevolent and meaningful, and the self as worthy. Specifically, previous assumptions about symptoms of PPD, childbirth and motherhood were formed within the context of the benevolent, meaningful, worthy paradigm. As we see, the sharp contrast of the reality of an untreated perinatal mood and anxiety disorder deconstructed women's reality, setting the stage for the onset of symptoms and devastating illness.

UNPREPARED FOR SYMPTOMS

The first common theme presented by the women in this study was a description of being unprepared for the onset of symptoms. Being unprepared was experienced as a sudden and distressing awareness of the symptoms of PPD, as Vicki described; "I just never had any idea of what depression was until it hit me the way it did. Everything was fine, and then it was just like, bam!"

When the symptoms occurred, women felt a sense of being caught off guard, shocked, helpless, and uncertain as to what was happening. The "before" dimension of the experience of transformation through PPD included the collision between the onset of symptoms and preconceptions of motherhood (see Figure 1). The underlying thread was that women were not given information regarding risk factors or symptoms in prenatal care. Care providers and childbirth educators failed to provide basic information on the existence of PPD altogether, much less risk factors, symptoms, or resources to recognize the reality of how those symptoms felt in real-time.

Not surprisingly, the onset of symptoms was a shock, as Morgan shared:

It took me completely by surprise. It took me by surprise because I didn't know what it was and why it happens to some and not others. When I was in my throes of postpartum depression, I just didn't know what was going on with me at all. I mean, no one had warned me about postpartum depression, I had no educational materials, and my OB/GYN never warned me about it. I didn't understand what it was.

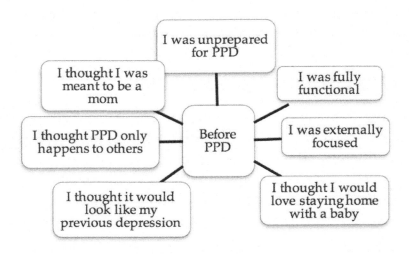

Fig 1: Representation of Symptoms Before PPD

Margery, who experienced postpartum psychosis as a result of severe generalized anxiety, stated,

> I wasn't prepared for it. No one ever told me about it even as a registered nurse. Knowing what I know now, I had several risk factors. And I went through undiagnosed, I feel like, postpartum depression and anxiety with both of my children. We had the assistance of a reproductive help with our first and then got unexpectedly pregnant with our second. And I'm pretty sure I had prenatal anxiety with my second. Even had heart palpitations and racing heart rate and got sent to the cardiologist and everything. But nobody ever brought up anxiety; was never mentioned.

Georgia's experience echoed a lack of preparation, such as care providers failing to discuss symptoms in prenatal care. Stephanie and Haley described the same thing.

> Nobody—my obstetrician, none of my obstetricians had ever mentioned postpartum depression or anything like that to me in any of my prenatal visits; they had never asked me about my history of any kind of mood or anxiety issues. They never brought it up in any way. **(Georgia)**

> I attended an eight-week childbirth class, and PPD was never mentioned once. **(Stephanie)**

> I took a birthing class. It was never discussed, other than a cursory thing. **(Haley)**

When prenatal providers failed to discuss, educate, or address PPD, women couldn't contextualize symptoms as related to the perinatal period, much less prepare for them. When the symptoms emerged, they were, therefore, not baby-related; they were something unknown, overwhelming, and frightening. As a result of the lack of preparation in the prenatal period, women did not realize they were struggling until symptoms became severe.

Still others, like Paula, did not realize what was happening until the symptoms presented within a context associated with life before the baby, such as work:

> *Everything was set, I was ready to go back to work, and then this just threw an entire curveball. I just wasn't prepared for the emotions and my anxiety, and it really kind of came to a head when I realized that I shouldn't be sitting in our lactation room crying every time I pump because that was the only place that I could let go.*

It is important to note the domino effect of fear here. The expression of not being prepared for a negative event and the sense of sudden and complete disorder resulted in a fear that left women questioning the safety of the world. These women experienced the onset of PPD as an unexpected injury. They didn't see it coming. They didn't know it was even a possibility, given no previous history of depression or anxiety. They could not believe that they were experiencing it. They had no concept of what it was or what to call it. Unprepared, in this context, meant women were unprotected and vulnerable, leading to the loss of the fundamental assumption of safety and invulnerability necessary for health and well-being.

Women with Histories of Depression or Anxiety

For those with no prior history of mood or anxiety disorders, the before dimension placed women at the nexus of profound ontological challenges: the previous assumptions about life before the baby and the reality of life as a new mother with symptoms of a mood or anxiety disorder.

Interestingly, women who had a history of depression or anxiety before the onset of PPD also reported feeling unprepared. There was a sense of disequilibrium between what symptoms of depression or anxiety felt like before PPD, and the lived experience of the symptoms of PPD.

> *I had already had depression issues for most of my, you know, from my teens through my adult years. So, I had been getting treated, you know, off and on since probably about age 15, for bouts of depression. But for most of that time, before I had my son, it really was depression and not anxiety, that was the problem. And so, I had been on and off SSRIs and things like that, and, you know, but basically stable. when my son's birth was so long and difficult, and it was, I felt like, "This is not what I was promised."* **(Deborah)**

> *I did have some depressive episodes in the past, so I thought I might have depression when my daughter was born. I had no idea, though, what that would look like, though. I thought it would look like my previous depression episodes of anxiety.* **(Janis)**

Previous coping strategies to manage symptoms of depression and anxiety either no longer worked or were no longer available due to the added responsibilities of new motherhood.

> *I didn't realize before I got PPD how many issues I actually had because my life just sort of functioned. I didn't have to have a child to worry about, and if I was OCD about something, it didn't really affect anybody. So, I like to say; I didn't realize how messed up I was until I actually got PPD.* **(Vicki)**

Previous Assumptions About Mental Illness

For others, previously formed negative beliefs about mental illness, or stereotypes about women who got PPD contributed to the experience of being unprepared. Prior assumptions of what PPD would look like contributed to confusion and shame regarding the experience of symptoms.

> *I had some very negative points of view on what postpartum depression was and I just kind of felt like, there are cases where it's really extreme, but there's a lot of people out there who are just having a hard time adjusting and maybe they didn't want the baby and, like, all these horrible thoughts — and now I cringe, thinking, oh my God, how could I have ever thought that?* **(Betsy)**

Preconceptions of how women should handle PPD contributed to shame, fear, and confusion when their symptoms developed. Morgan explained that before she got PPD, "I thought PPD was mind over matter, and I would not let myself succumb to it." These thoughts and beliefs about the symptoms and the experience of getting through it contributed to a startling disconnect between previous perceptions of themselves, the reality of becoming ill, and expectational beliefs about the postpartum period. When women became ill, they could no longer recognize who they were, as Morgan described:

> *I went from a highly functioning, multitasking individual with X number of years of work experience, to someone who couldn't sleep, couldn't eat, and suffered from panic attacks.* **(Morgan)**

The ontological split between beliefs about motherhood and the reality of postpartum depression shattered an assumption of the world as making sense. Each day, the mothers described expecting to see the mother they thought they would be, and never seeing it. Women never saw themselves function as the mothers they believed they would be before PPD, and it shattered their assumptions of self as worthy. In the broader context of social norms of motherhood, a shattered assumption of self as worthy to mother added insult to injury for many women.

Previous Assumptions About Motherhood

Powerful social, cultural, and familial messages about idealized motherhood and created preconceptions that motherhood would be instinctive, effortless, and immediate. As the feminist poet Adrienne Rich (1986/1976) noted,

> Motherhood—unmentioned in the histories of conquest and serfdom, wars and treaties, exploration and imperialism—has a history, it has an ideology; it is more fundamental than tribalism or nationalism (p. 33).

The historical, social, and cultural constructs of motherhood exist. The myth of motherhood embeds itself in the fabric of our social structure, despite all practical evidence. As feminist philosopher Sara Ruddick (1995) stated, "Mothers are no more—and no less—blessed with stamina and gifted in courage than other women and men" (p. 112). We carry powerful, yet invisible intergenerational beliefs and prejudices about motherhood with us *into* motherhood.

These beliefs mingle with our personal experience and are used as comparative schemas. We judge ourselves against the dominant ideals of motherhood. We bend to it, often inauthentically, as if gearing up for a rite of passage with the utmost honor, import, and significance. Plus, if we get it wrong, in the eyes of society, it's game over. Under what Ruddick (1995) called "the gaze of others" (p. 112), our legitimacy as reproductive women is continuously scrutinized, and our foundational assumptions of ourselves as worthy is destroyed.

The media is definitely a part of it. I will say that I got some messaging from my mother, too, that ended up really adding to my pain in the end. I felt like the message I got was, "You're made to do this, and you'll know what to do when the time comes." Which, I guess, is true to a certain extent, but also kind of lays pressure on that I think is a little bit undue. I just got the sense of the mom is supposed to know what to do right away, is supposed to enjoy every second, is supposed to remember that these days are precious. And that your boobs will be the comfort for the baby, your body will know what to do, and that it will be this beautiful, seamless experiences.

There was a lot of learning involved for me, and there was a lot of saying, "Oh, not all motherhood looks one way," and, "Oh, you're supposed to want to stay home with your kids, and you're supposed to cry and weep when you have to go back to work. You're supposed to never want anybody else to be with them but you." And it just is not that way for me, and it's definitely not been that way for a few people close to me. **(Deborah)**

I think people just don't want to see it because everyone wants you, you know they want to see you as, like, you're a normal, happy, glowing postpartum person. And everyone's so concerned about the baby and focused on the baby, you know, as they should be to some degree; it's just—it is, I mean, I don't know what the answer is but it's, like, really, I think it's a really bad thing. **(Adrienne)**

I had this idealistic picture of the way being a parent should be . . . it was, like, way over the top. **(Mindy)**

The expectations that I had internalized throughout my life as a woman, what a mother is supposed to be, what society shows you they expect from a mother, in a woman, expectations of myself just to do the best possible job taking care of my children. I'm very type-A personality, very conscientious, very observant person, which I was all those things before, obviously. But this was a heightened state of all of that, to the point where it ended up almost destroying me, not asking for help and really having that expectation from all around or wherever it comes from that we're supposed to do this on our own. **(Heather)**

I was not the mom I thought I would be, caring for a newborn, not liking it, etc. You have so many other dreams and images of what you're going to be like with a newborn, and I wasn't any of those things. **(Betsy)**

I thought I was meant to be a mom. **(Stephanie)**

I am the oldest on both sides of my parent's families, and I was always the one that babysat and took care of all the kids. I always had a kid on my hip. And so, for me, to feel the way I did about my own baby scared the hell out of me. **(Faith)**

I felt very prepared for having a baby. I had been an older sister and a babysitter from the time I was little, and a preschool teacher. And so, I felt like motherhood was going to be a very natural thing for me and just expected completely for it to be a good experience. I mean, just hearing my child cry inconsolably, that's very triggering to hear a child. And that happens a lot with babies! And you can't always calm them down or fix it. And so, it's, like, wow, you know, no one told me when I had a baby that I'm going to be triggered a lot. **(Skye)**

I really had this whole philosophy of "I was going to breastfeed and cloth diaper and co-sleep and un-school." Like not even like traditional homeschool, no, I'm going to go totally rogue un-school. Before you had your children, you thought you would want to do those kinds of things. I mean, I was a child specialist. I worked with abused children: play therapy. That's what I went to grad school for is like family therapy, play therapy, a child specialist. I really believed, "it'll be great. I'll be great with kids." I don't know why it never occurred to me before I had kids that I would be unhappy staying at home with them. It had never occurred to me that I am someone who would not be happy at home with children all day. **(Beatrice)**

The repetition of "never occurred to me" underscores the lack of preparation for PPD. For someone to be a child specialist, have her own child, and then experience a completely different self, weakened her assumptions that the world made sense and that she was worthy of being a mother. My sense of Beatrice's experience was of someone having just trying to regain orientation in an unfamiliar world. This disconnect between constructs of motherhood before PPD and the reality of the experience, combined with no prenatal education about PPD, created an overall disequilibrium. Women were stunned by what was occurring, as the symptoms took hold. In effect, when symptoms did occur, women did not recognize them as PPD, and they did not recognize themselves as they did before.

Georgia's story further captures how PPD shattered assumptions:

When I graduated from college, the younger girls in my sorority wrote us these little books with impressions of us as the seniors. Mine said a lot of things about how confident I was, and how they all knew I was going to go on to do great things. During my PPD, I remember reading that book and thinking, "This book can't be written for me, because I don't recognize this person at all."

As we have seen, the core beliefs we hold about ourselves and the world frame our behavior in that world. The cognitive representations, mental templates of symbolic meaning, emotion, and efficacy or agency in the world guide our behavior.

UNPREPARED FOR TRAUMATIC CHILDBIRTH

The psychological disequilibrium caused by untreated PPD resulted in extreme, debilitating fear. For many, that fear was exacerbated by traumatic childbirth. In the first version of this book, I purposely did not speak to the prevalence of birth trauma in the sample, as I wanted to focus specifically on women's lived experience of untreated PPD. However, this version speaks to a broader range of experiences, including traumatic childbirth. To truly bring authenticity to the discussion, my own traumatic childbirth with Ziggy not only informs my view as a survivor but drives me to speak to the prevalence and correlation between perinatal mood and anxiety disorders and traumatic childbirth.

The theory I propose in this book is that the experience of untreated PPD, or any perinatal mood or anxiety disorder, is an experience of trauma and should be discussed as a traumatic life event. It no longer serves the discussion to compartmentalize traumatic birth from trauma as a result of PPD. The perinatal experience for a woman includes the full range of physical and the psychological—as she describes it. In the cases of 20 of the 25 women interviewed for this book, the perinatal experience included a traumatic childbirth.

I felt like motherhood was going to be a very natural thing for me and just expected completely for it to be a good experience. When I had the baby, everything went really well until after I delivered. I was able to have the baby completely as expected. I had a natural birth, and I had a wonderful gynecologist or OB who was very supportive and let me go natural as much as I wanted. But then after I gave birth to the baby, I had kind of a scary experience where I was hemorrhaging, and they almost had to take me and do some sort of emergency procedure. I think that may have been the start of things not being quite as good for me because that was scary and pretty painful and upsetting right after I had given birth when I just wanted to be able to hold my baby and enjoy my baby. I wasn't able to at all.

My husband had him across the room, and I could see them while people were pushing on me and trying to start an IV and doing all kinds of things. But that actually ended up okay. The bleeding did stop. After that, I roomed in with my baby. I remember just being really exhausted after having the baby. I wasn't prepared for how physically exhausted I would be. Also, I had torn pretty badly during birth, and so I wasn't prepared for the amount of pain that I was going to be in for the next two to four weeks. I did not expect that at all. **(Skye)**

It certainly was a traumatic birth, and in terms of he came very fast, he was an eleven-pound baby, it was very physical and different labor than I had envisioned. I certainly never envisioned his heart rate dropping and me losing a lot of blood, and he physically had to almost literally be torn from me to save him and all of those things, and not being able to hold him after he was born and all of those things. **(Anna)**

I had four units of blood taken or lost and replaced. And so, I was physically at a disadvantage and emotionally at a disadvantage. **(Morgan)**

During my birth, I did end up becoming preeclamptic, and I actually became eclamptic, and I had two seizures. During the seizures, it felt like I died; like, I'm pretty positive I died. I remember feeling, I remember my vision like splitting in half when the midwife was giving me fluid. After I seized, I remember trying to sit up because I felt like if I could sit up, I could breathe better and control what was happening to my body better. That's when an ambulance came to take me to the hospital. **(Karen)**

I planned a home birth, and I wanted one more than anything in the world. I labored for three days and had to have a caesarean. And it was a hard way to enter motherhood. And I felt like I had already failed at being a mom. **(Jamie)**

I had contractions on and off for a week before and then (inaudible) early in the morning, very early in the morning the day she was born, and we went—my husband and I went up to the hospital twice, once around five or six in the morning and we were sent home. We were very close to the hospital within ten minutes. I was so exhausted; I had been up since two in the morning. They gave me Ambien.

We were sent home, and then we went again midafternoon, sent home again because I wasn't dilated much. I laid down to try and sleep, and all of a sudden I started to feel the need to push and—I just started to push and I'm lying in my bed at home, my husband was about to leave to go to the grocery store; I caught him as he was walking out the door and I said, "I'm pushing; you need to call the doctor."

The Ambien had kicked in by then, so I don't remember the car ride to the hospital. I don't remember arriving at the hospital. He told me that I was pushing in the car, that he thought that we were—he was going to have to pull over and I was going to have the baby in the car or on the way up to the birthing unit. We got to the hospital, and I pushed for maybe 15 or 20 more minutes, and she was born. **(Janis)**

It was my second childbirth. I did not have this same experience with my first childbirth. My first child, I had an epidural when I got to seven centimeters. But with my second, I had a natural childbirth. When I was nine centimeters, and there was no going back, and I had no drugs, no epidural. I think that was a component of it because I entered into the pain of childbirth consciously. I had experienced trauma in my childhood. I feel like it brought me to places within myself that I had learned to defend against. **(Callie)**

Even though I had a great pregnancy, he was breech at the end. And so, going from thinking I was going to have a typical birth and then finding out I was going to have to have a planned C-section because the baby was breech was really devastating for me. Physically, everything went fine, but I was not doing well. I had symptoms, and nobody was asking me about it. It was like I had felt like I was in this tunnel vision in the last month of my pregnancy. The day he was born, I couldn't sleep and felt like this can't be happening, you know, just a little bit disconnected from what was actually going on. Knowing what I know now, I think I really just looked at it as being sad. I mean, I expressed that sadness to people and told my husband how I was not excited about having to have a C-section and things being changed in a way I wasn't planning for or happy to have changed in that way. **(Grace)**

It felt like this black curtain just, like, went over me the second I delivered my son. I mean, it was crazy. And you know, I had experienced depression before, but it was, like, slow-moving, mild; I could still function. This was, like, the scariest feeling I had ever felt in my life. I remember thinking to myself, maybe I'm having some weird reaction to the epidural. I didn't know what was going on. **(Betsy)**

CONCLUSION

Functioning while not functioning, remembering and not remembering, birthing and possibly dying, expecting and the delivery of the unexpected. Myriad contradictions in the before dimension of PPD explain how being unprepared for PPD lost the necessary assumptions forming the theory of theories (Epstein, 1980): that the world is safe, it makes sense, and that we are worthy of it.

This chapter described the process of transforming through PPD began with an ending—an ending of all that was known before—cracking the foundational and necessary assumption of the self as worthy in the role of mother. In the next chapter, women describe the experience shock, fear, and disorientation caused by lack of preparation. The result of untreated PPD is a shattering of the assumptions about the world as benevolent and meaningful at the hands of an untreated postpartum mood or anxiety disorder.

CHAPTER 3

DURING POSTPARTUM DEPRESSION: SHATTERED ASSUMPTIONS

Who gives birth? And to whom is it given?
Certainly, it doesn't feel like giving, which implies
a flow, a gentle handing over, no coercion . . . Maybe
the phrase was made by someone viewing the result
only . . . yet one more thing that needs to be renamed.
– **Margaret Atwood,** *The Blind Assassin*

This chapter illustrates that women were transformed through untreated PPD because it deconstructed their fundamental beliefs in the safety and sanity of the world, resulting in terror. The lived experience of physical and psychological symptoms of untreated PPD is described. In the wake of being unprepared for when symptoms developed, women were confused, disoriented, and terrified of what they were experiencing.

PHYSICAL SYMPTOMS: THE BODY OFFLINE

Recovering from birth while experiencing a mood or anxiety disorder impacted the body directly, quickly, and drastically. Physical pain, loss of appetite, agitation, and insomnia were pervasive. The experience of physical pain or a sense of physical injury and wounding was thematic (see Figure 2).

Physical Pain

It physically felt painful. I—my heart raced, and my chest felt tight. I had a horrible lump in my throat, and I physically hurt from the emotions. I just remember feeling almost physical pain from the depression of it all and the anxiety. (**Anna**)

I remember telling my husband, "I don't remember any time I wasn't in pain because the surgery hurt, the labor hurt, breastfeeding hurt, recovery hurt, and I was just like I'm just a bag of hurt." (**Jamie**)

Appetite

The loss of appetite and rapid weight loss was also noted physical components of PPD.

When I was depressed with postpartum depression, I physically could not even stand the thought of eating, and I lost weight quickly. It was pretty alarming, actually. (**Morgan**)

I wasn't eating very well. I would pretty much only eat things that I could just throw in the microwave and warm up. I wasn't cooking anymore. And, you know, at the time, I don't think I recognized it at all as depression. I think I just felt like I was just so overwhelmed with the baby. (**Skye**)

I could never relax because I always felt that I was on call. And it was my sole responsibility to keep this human being alive, which is not a small thing, to put it mildly. So, at that point, my husband really started to notice. I told him I wasn't eating. I was dropping weight very quickly. I got back down to my pre-pregnancy weight very fast at that point. (**Adrienne**)

Insomnia

In addition to pain and loss of appetite, a significant physical component of the experience of PPD was insomnia.

I had several nights of just not sleeping. I just sat in the nursing rocker and had the baby. She slept, and I nursed on and off, and I watched the clock. I was absolutely exhausted. **(Janis)**

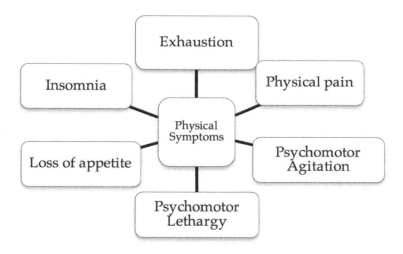

Fig 2: Representation of the Physical Components of PPD

It started out not being able to fall asleep, then not sleeping at all. And it went on for nine days. I don't have any more anxiety or depression. I just still can't sleep solid through the night. But I know one day, hopefully soon, it will come. **(Sienna)**

The experience of insomnia for a woman suffering from PPD gets lost in the general understanding of lack of sleep for new mothers. It's important to note the difference between. When women with PPD experience insomnia, they describe not sleeping, even when tired and the baby sleeps.

As I shared in the Introduction, I went for nearly three weeks without any sleep. It felt as if my ability to sleep was broken. Early evening brought extreme anxiety, heart palpitations, dizziness, and nausea. When nighttime came, and I would have usually been sleeping and could not, the anxiety grew. During the day, my energy didn't relent. I was wired and tired 24/7.

Physical Fatigue/Agitation

Along with insomnia, the body responds to PPD with other physical symptoms such as agitation or extreme lethargy, or both. This is called psychomotor lethargy. Vicki describes it this way; *"I couldn't get out of bed, I couldn't shower, I couldn't function."* It can also manifest with a sense of physical restlessness, as Paula describes; *"Physically, not being able to sit still. I felt like I always had to be doing something."* Helena described the relentlessness of physical exhaustion.

> *I was always tired. I couldn't sleep. I couldn't eat. I couldn't do my basic needs. And yet, I was expected to kind of run this marathon of motherhood through this gauntlet of arrows coming at me and boulders coming at me. I felt like I was running with sprained ankles, and gashes, and just all these things, and I could never heal, I could never catch my breath.* (**Helena**)

> *I just remember coming home from that hospital and waking up in the morning was the hardest thing to do. It just felt like I just couldn't even get out of bed and bear to face the pain. Walking down the stairs was terrifying.* (**Callie**)

The relentlessness of the physical symptoms of PPD revealed a component of untreated PPD as potentially traumatic. Women describe extreme physical discomfort that doesn't end. The experience of the symptoms not ending is worded with the language of terror.

In 2000, after Ziggy was born, my provider told me to take 50 mg of Benadryl to sleep. When it didn't work, I was terrified. That much Benadryl would have knocked me out for two days before I had PPD. When the treatment prescribed by my physician did not work, I was even more convinced that I would never be fixed. With no reference as to what was occurring, or how to understand physical symptoms of PPD within reasonable range of postpartum physical adjustments, the fact that the prescribed cure wasn't working manifested extreme and pervasive fear. I was terrified, constantly.

The experience of that kind of pervasive terror is all-consuming. Similar to Sienna's not being able to catch her breath, my physical symptoms of PPD felt like constantly inhaling. Imagine only being able to inhale while witnessing yourself come closer and closer to an edge of life, not knowing if you will ever exhale. Now imagine doing so while holding a newborn baby. That experience is fear on steroids; it barely even resembles fear. It is the limbic system in overdrive—amygdala and hypothalamus looping distress signals to the body to stop what it was doing and prepare for the worst.

The peripheral functions of the body are logged off, no time to feel hunger or sleep. The heart pumps faster, the adrenal glands pump cortisol, and directions are sent from the thalamus to shut down frontal lobe activity of problem-solving, concentration, abstract thinking, and regulated emotional response. In this kind of terror, women are left to the mercy of the reptilian brain evolved from ancestors—the body reacts with complete system shut down. Fight, flight, or freeze is no joke. It is a living death.

PSYCHOLOGICAL SYMPTOMS: BRAIN OFFLINE

The terror experienced because of the collapsing down brought by physical symptoms of untreated PPD was compounded by the experience of frightening psychological symptoms that included feeling disconnected from others, hypervigilance, intrusive thoughts, suicidal ideation, and psychosis.

Disconnected

Women described the experience of a disconnection from the world around them as a severing of sense of self in relation to time, space, and responsiveness to emotional cues.

> I was about six weeks out . . . the explanation or the moment I was telling you about, during childbirth, when I had that everything-happening moment; it was kind of like pulsing. But I was still in this kind of numb place, I would say. And it was about six weeks after my son was born that I was outside with my son and my two and a half-year old. And it was a beautiful sunny day, and that's when it hit me because I'm a big nature person; it was something about that moment, recognizing, I felt so disconnected from . . . you know, it really did, like I described depression, seemed like a gray cloud.

> I was so disconnected from myself, or, no, not from myself, from the beautiful weather around me: the sunshine, the puffy clouds, the blue sky. It just hit me in that moment, and I was terrified. I was losing my mind. Like, I literally was so deep inside of myself and the recognition of how deep I was, was terrifying. And I didn't know how I was going to get back.

> And that's when the moment of that real recognition on the ground level. I think I had already recognized it on a spiritual level, but this

was the real, you know, ground level. And the anxiety at that point became, you know, prior to that, there was some, you know, different emotions coming up, but I wasn't really embodying them, and I was rationalizing it and still pushing it away as, "You know, this is nothing. This isn't a big deal. This is baby blues." But in that moment, it was like, "Nope; there was none of that." It was like, "Holy shit, where am I?" And this place is terrifying because I was just in it. And I saw the truth emotionally of where I was. **(Callie)**

Callie's story depicts the sense of profound fear as a result of her disconnection from her world due to untreated PPD. During PPD, women lived with emotions, thoughts, and realities that they did not understand. Not understanding these symptoms contributed to the constant sense of terror and sadness (see Figure 3).

Uncontrollable Crying

Sadness was described by women as the experience of uncontrollable crying.

I was crying every day with him, all day. I couldn't stop crying. **(Jamie)**

Sometimes, when the baby would cry, and I would cry. I would just sit there and cry with him because I didn't know what to do. **(Skye)**

I literally could not stop crying. I remember thinking about how I could possibly not be like dying of dehydration because everything I drank just came out in tears. It was just constant. **(Betsy)**

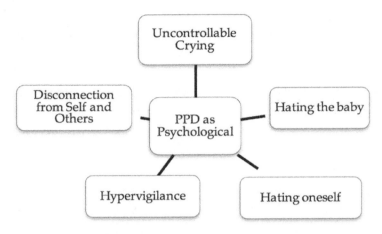

Fig 3: Representation of the Psychological Components of PPD

Think about the last time you cried. Now imagine that you couldn't stop even after the situation had resolved. The emotional trigger causing the reaction ends, and you keep crying. A kind of involuntary leaking, like the stomach flu. For these women, not being able to control crying was frightening, psychologically distressing. Notice how Georgia's description of crying demonstrates a shift in the description from symptoms of sadness, to symptoms of distress and trauma.

> *I was definitely in triage mode after my first son was born. I came home from my first doctor's appointment following birth, and I just sobbed and sobbed and sobbed and sobbed. And of course, I didn't know at the time that that wasn't, kind of, a "normal reaction" to that.* **(Georgia)**

Similarly, Vicki recounted a social event during which she experienced uncontrollable crying as traumatic.

> *We went to dinner the night before for my husband's birthday, and I cried through the whole dinner. I cried at how I destroyed our lives. It was very traumatic, and I still remember it to a T. I can't*

remember anything about my son's early months, but I can remember my postpartum to a T, and it was very, very traumatic. **(Vicki)**

Hypervigilance

In addition, uncontrollable crying, women described pervasive hyperarousal or hypervigilance. For example, Deborah shared,

> *It was, like, hypervigilance, like, to the nth degree. I never experienced the feeling—like I had never been put in the position to be responsible for the life of another person before. All of a sudden, I was acutely aware that if I didn't do the right thing, my baby could get sick. If I didn't do the right thing, he could die. If I didn't do the right thing then, you know, what if I drop him? What if I do this? What if I did and it was just, like, not normal. It was overwhelming, and I was afraid to be alone with him a lot.*

> *And it was, sort of, contrasted by the fact that my husband was a natural from, like, day one. The cries didn't bother him; the needing to walk him for hours and hours didn't bother him. He was just like, "Nope, this is being dad, I got it. Like, we're good." It was helpful, but it was also exacerbating how alone I felt with all of the feelings of, "I'm supposed to be a natural at this, and I'm not, and he is, and why don't I feel the bond? And why don't I feel like I can handle this? How could a little person be so scary, basically?" But I felt a lot in those first really early, especially the newborn days, that I was gritting my teeth through the whole thing. There were no violins; it was really hard.* **(Deborah)**

"There were no violins." Deborah's story presents an experience of a split between the ideal motherhood and the reality of relentless hypervigilance. Again, the experience of not being able to control the ending of an affective state when the cause for cognitive concern passed was in and of itself frightening. It was as if something was broken in the brain.

Paula echoed an experience of hypervigilant thoughts concerning her baby. Her description expressed the distress and the difficulty articulating the depth of the distress.

> *I worried about everything, what the girls ate, how they were doing . . . I couldn't really articulate how I was feeling, but I knew I wasn't going to hurt—they ask, like, the basic questions, really trying to assess was I in any type of crisis, and at that time, no, but I knew I wasn't feeling right.* **(Paula)**

For Skye, an ongoing sense of worry pervaded her thoughts.

> *I just couldn't shake the feeling that something was going to go wrong. I felt very much disconnected from the baby. I remember kind of looking at him and just not feeling much of anything; it was almost like I was looking at someone else's baby.* **(Skye)**

Women were both aware of their symptoms and horrified by them.

> *I thought I was a horrible mom. I couldn't understand the thoughts I was having. I really just chalked it up to being tired.* **(Mindy)**

> *I didn't really feel like I should be around because I thought whatever was wrong with me was contagious in some way.* **(Betsy)**

> *At about three months or so, I started to really get obsessed about his sleeping and making sure that he slept enough, and his eating. I never stopped keeping track of his feeding schedule. He was up every two to three hours, and, of course, not taking a bottle. He needed me during those times. That really set it off for me. Within about a couple of weeks, I really realized the irritability had*

transformed into a rage for me. That was very surprising, confusing, frightening. **(Adrienne)**

Intrusive Thoughts

Psychological symptoms manifested as disorienting cognitive patterns of terrifying intrusive thoughts and a sense of split with reality. Note the language similarities between Anna's and Sandy's experiences of some of their most severe symptoms.

My eyes didn't look like me, my face; I didn't look like myself at all. I did not feel like myself. I felt like this other person had taken over my body because the thoughts I was having and the reactions I was having were just so unlike myself. There is so much not trusting yourself and not feeling like yourself and kind of feeling like the real you is kind of watching all of this take place." **(Anna)**

I remember staring at myself in the mirror and thinking, "That's not me in the mirror." And it didn't look like me in the mirror. When I went into the OB's office, it was like my body was in the chair, but I was watching myself from above. I totally disconnected that day. I slid downhill pretty fast that day. I wasn't myself. This is not normal. This is not me. **(Sandy)**

I had fallen asleep one night, and my husband was holding our son and sleeping on the bed the hospital provided for him. I had fallen asleep, and when I woke up I realized there had been like many hours that I had fallen asleep, and I hadn't heard the baby, I hadn't fed the baby in quite a long time, and so, like, I got myself out of bed. This is, you know, post-C-section, and I walked over to them, and when I looked down, he had a really peaceful, still look on his face. And when I looked at it, I thought he was dead. When I looked at him, I thought he was dead. And my first thought was that he was dead. And then my second thought was that I was like, "Oh gosh, I don't have to do this."

You know, I was overwhelmed with the thought of having to parent him, and like the weight of that, my life has changed in this way even though I wanted it so badly. In the hospital, nobody actually asked me how I was doing in that way. Then I started to have an anxiety attack before I went home. I told my husband about it that I was feeling anxious and, you know, and we talked through it, like, maybe it's just going home and all those things. But then when I got home, then I proceeded to have, like, panic attacks every day for a long time. And yeah, so, we knew right away that something wasn't right." **(Grace)**

I had intrusive thoughts of throwing my son against the wall, which I never admitted to anyone because I was horrified and ashamed that I could even have those pop into my head. I was terrified to be alone. I remember white-knuckling and driving down the road and having those intrusive thoughts. **(Callie)**

It felt like I hated her a lot of the time. Like I hated the baby. And when people would say, "Oh, she's so cute," I would nod and pretend, but I didn't really feel like that inside. **(Stephanie)**

I never, in all three of my experiences, never felt like I wanted to hurt them. I just didn't want anything to do with them because I was terrified of them. I was clueless, completely clueless. **(Faith)**

Karen's story revealed a pattern of speech I would note in the language of many women as they started to describe the most difficult elements of their experience of untreated PPD.

I started hallucinating. I was so fearful that if I moved, I was going to die that I couldn't move . . . It was like I had a panic attack so bad that I couldn't move. And so, I got admitted to the hospital by my parent's house. (**Karen**)

Notice the long pause in Karen's sentence indicated by the ellipses, where Karen stopped talking in the interview. Silence. She paused for several moments before she finished telling me that she ended up hospitalized for her hallucinations. This speech pattern mirrored the lived experience of severe PPD symptoms: the language of questioning, repeating, pausing, slowing, losing track of the subject of the sentence. For example, note Vicki's description.

I remember the first time we wanted to pick up a pizza, and we went to jump in the car together, and it was like, "I can't go? I can't go. No, I have to stay here with the baby. I just can't get in the car and go?" And that was actually the night my postpartum started. It was the night after Christmas. We went to get takeout. I realized I couldn't go, and it was just, "My God, I can't go. I can't get in the car with him and go." (**Vicki**)

Vicki repeated "can't go" six times in that passage. The repetition signaled a cognitive loop referencing a particularly distressing event. Something as simple as realizing she could not get in the car and go for pizza the way she had many times before—shattered her understanding of the world. As her PPD progressed, Vicki's thoughts became more extreme. As she told me this, her sentences filled with more repetitions, broken by pauses, and patterns of stopping and starting.

Constantly, I would constantly just tell my husband, "Oh, let's give him up for adoption. He's a blonde hair, blue-eyed boy, he's . . . someone's going to snatch him up in a minute." And my husband would always say to me, "Let's give it a year; let's see how you feel in a year." . . . So, I was convinced when that year was up, we were giving him up, we were going to give him up for adoption.

I ended up basically suicidal. I had a lot of suicidal thoughts, driving my car into a tree, and if I wasn't going to do that, I was going to move to Florida, and my girlfriend lives there. I was going to get a job at her restaurant, and just start my life over. **(Vicki)**

Suicidal Ideation

The frequency of reports of suicidal ideation was an unexpected finding. There was nothing in my research design nor my screening questions about suicidal ideation. The prevalence of thoughts of suicide in the sample of 25 women was that 22 (88%) reported having intrusive thoughts of self-harm, suicidal ideation, or desire to leave, and 19 (76%) reported experiencing PPD as life-threatening. While the sample size is small, the high prevalence of intrusive thoughts of ending one's life was startling, given the range of experience, location, and background of 25 women.

Knowing that the majority of women had dealt with thoughts of suicide gave credence to what I would then uncover in their stories. Women minimized suicidal ideation in their language.

I didn't experience self-harm, feeling my biggest things were just wanting to leave. And, you know, I had, like, a plan for my new life, and I knew my husband and my son would never forgive me, but it was going to be okay because I would feel better even though then knowing I wouldn't feel better.

I think my biggest thing was that I just, like, the thought. I mean, when you're going through an anxiety attack or going through depression, your thoughts tell you, like, "This is never going to end," right? And just having that feeling of, like, "I can't. I can't live like this," like, this is like, "I can't do this like this. I have to, like, try everything to make this go away."

Like, they're not . . . Like, I was willing to take any medication that they would give me. I knew even though they wouldn't give me anything, and I just wanted the feelings to stop, you know? I wanted to be able to, like, to feel the feelings that people tell you that you magically feel when you have a baby. I didn't get to feel any of those feelings, and I wanted that, you know? I would rather feel than what I was feeling. So, I think that's what really guided me is just that intense urge just to make it stop. **(Grace)**

I didn't have thoughts of harming myself or suicidal ideation. I had this constant stream of thoughts, though, where I mentioned, I just need to go away, I need to run away. I can't do this anymore. This is not the life I want. It's not the life I thought was going to happen. I made a mistake. I ruined our lives by having a second baby and bringing all of this chaos. So, for me, I don't know why it didn't lean in that manner of suicidal ideations or thoughts of hurting myself. I know that we're all chemically different. So, perhaps that part of it, and perhaps I got treatment before it went that way with the continuum. I just wanted to walk away from this life. **(Adrienne)**

I really felt like dying, not like to an attempt level of suicidality, but just definitely a latent level of suicidality. **(Beatrice)**

I became, I would say, mildly suicidal. I didn't actually take any steps, but I had the full prescription of my antidepressant and kind of sat there calculating, "If I take all of this, would it be enough to kill me or will it just be enough to maybe cause irreparable harm to the baby and then I'll have to live with that for the rest of my life?" **(Dana)**

"Mildly suicidal" while having a plan to complete suicide indicates a minimization of the severity of despair. As women shared their suicidal thoughts, the details were precise, but the gravity was downplayed. Here is Sienna's description,

Every night, I would tell my husband to take me to the hospital because I didn't want to live. I was taking my Zoloft. The doctor prescribed me, at one point, Ambien and Ativan, which didn't work. And I also had pain meds from my delivery, and I also had trazadone, and I would want to take all of them because I wanted to sleep so bad, but I didn't want to die, so I knew, in the back of my head, I didn't want to die so I would give my husband the pills after I took them at night and say, "Hide these." And that's what we did for probably a good month. **(Sienna)**

Diana's experience also involved thoughts of overdose.

I went to one psychiatrist, and his answer—he was very old-school—he just wanted to give me new prescriptions every week. So, my medications were changing every single week. He was giving me all these, like, ones that made me totally out of it, and I was taking them, and then I just had it. One night, I called my sister—she lived down the street. And I said, "That's it, I'm taking my all medicine, I'm done." And she came down, and I went into a mental hospital for, I think it was nine days. I was definitely suicidal.

I don't know if I—if my sister hadn't had shown up like right down the street, then I probably would have taken a handful of pills, yeah, for sure. But I didn't, I didn't get that far because she got there. My sister and my mom were like, "I don't understand. We just did it. We just got through being a mom. You've got to just do it." And I was like, "I'm trying to just do it." I tried "fake it until you make it" as long as I could. And I was getting it done, but I sure did want to die. **(Diana)**

Did you catch it? If I hadn't transcribed the interview, I might have missed it myself. Underneath the description of events, underneath all of the words, *"I sure did want to die."*

Descriptions revealed deep and pervasive desperation to end the suffering of the symptoms of untreated PPD permanently. A disturbing trend in language was that women wanted to choose a method that would result in completed suicide. Several women discussed violent ideations of self-harm, as Paula and Anna described.

I did suffer from intrusive thoughts. They were pretty horrible. Most of mine involved me falling down the stairs or getting into a car accident. **(Paula)**

My lowest moment was probably when I was in the car by myself, and I thought, very rationally, that the oncoming Mack truck that I should turn in front of it and that way, I wouldn't be a burden to my family, who was in such pain watching me suffer. **(Anna)**

Women explained how their thought processes around suicide included motivation for finality. Importantly, women specifically noted that they didn't so much want to die, as they wanted PPD to end. Nevertheless, the plans made for completion were significant, as in the case of Georgia.

One night, I was lying in bed, and I thought—my apartment building was seven stories high. I thought, if I go up and jump off the roof, I don't know if I'll die because I didn't know if seven stories were high enough to actually kill myself. I thought, "I definitely don't want to be a vegetable." If I'm going to do this, like, I need to die. I didn't see any—I didn't want to die, I just really wanted to sleep. I just wanted everything to stop. I couldn't, and I just couldn't handle it anymore. So finally, that next morning, I went to my husband and said, "I thought about throwing myself off of the building last night, and I have no idea what's going on with me." **(Georgia)**

As Georgia and others described, wanting to die was, in and of itself, a life-threatening experience of symptoms during untreated

PPD. As close as women got to acting, with plans and access to means of completing suicide, only two attempts were reported.

Perhaps it's the intimacy of suicide that shields us from acknowledging its stark gravity. The privacy of suicidal thoughts insulates us from exposure to stigma and judgment. Stigma, especially stigma of the mentally ill new mother, muffles our explicit expressions of wanting to die.

Our own internalized stigma and fear of separation from the central reason for living, our baby, pull us into invisible, punishing, and provocative thoughts. My own experience of suicidal ideation postpartum was paradoxical. Ending my life preoccupied with my thoughts while emotionally, my love for my precious baby boy grew. It was an experience of feeling both essential to his life and a risk to his future happiness all at once.

In some ways, suicidal ideation is like having hives. The relentless silent screams of the skin itching, pulling our attention to a basic reflex to scratch—to end the sensation, only to have the itch occur elsewhere, everywhere, endlessly. In this way, intrusive, involuntary thoughts of harming oneself fester, fueling a growing urgent need to act, to react in irrational extraordinary ways, just to end the suffering because of the symptoms.

Intrusive Thoughts of Harming Others

Ego dystonic are known as symptoms of severe mood and anxiety disorders.

The day I ended up getting hospitalized, I woke up that morning, and I had silent little voices in my head. I wouldn't say that I had psychosis, but I was heading towards a psychotic break. I had little voices in my head that just whisper, "Let go. Just let go because you can't do this anymore. You're tired, just let go and if you just take a pillow and . . ."

Every time I walked by my daughter's room that day, it was really tempting to get a pillow. Once it started getting really overpowering, I just went into our bedroom, closed the door, curled up on the bed, called my then-husband, and I was like, "I need you to come home." I had the overwhelming urge to actually act, and thank God, right before, I knew this wasn't right. I remember rocking back and forth and saying, "I just don't want to be Andrea Yates. Just don't let me be Andrea Yates." I remember that day very, very clearly. **(Sandy)**

Margery's Story

So, it's just a perfect storm of, I guess, for it to happen. Throughout the day, I did things that were completely outside of my normal. I went and quit work. Called my boss. I was, like, "I'm done," which was not like me. I was driving, which is very scary to think that I was not in my right mind to be driving around.

I called a woman who I met with the night before at the prayer meeting, and she worked at the Children's department during the day. I told her, "Please," I said, "Please check on the pastor. The children will be okay." . . . Because I thought this pastor was going to die. I think I texted her, and I never got a response. I went and checked on the pastor myself, which is not like me. I went and had a conversation with him, came home, apparently quoted scriptures to my husband that he never thought I would memorize. It all just seemed very, very real to me. I thought that the pastor was going to die, and my husband was supposed to take his place.

It was Memorial Day weekend, and I was supposed to drive myself with my kids to the beach by myself. But at that point, I thought Jesus was returning. I'm pretty sure my kids were asleep. I grabbed them up, and I said, "Please, save me. Please, save my children. Please, save our friends."

I don't think I've really told many people this, but at that moment, I could see, like, almost a difference in my children, like, almost laughing at me. It was bizarre. Almost like, I don't even want to say the devil, but they were laughing at me. My husband came back in the room, and he's like, "What are you doing?" I'm like, "I'm praying," and he said I was white as a ghost.

He called 911. When they came, and I was telling them to pump on my chest because I thought I was going to die. I was passing out and coming back and passing out and coming back. I felt like I was watching myself from, like, from above. They took me to the ambulance, and I got in, and I got back out. I was, like, "I'm fine. I do not need to go with you guys." There were people there that my husband called to watch the kids. I remember their faces. Like, "What are you doing in here?" Like, "I'm fine, y'all can go."

So, my husband had to ride in the back of the ambulance with me. We went to the ER. I spent three nights in a psychiatric ER. We were 45 minutes away from a mother-baby unit at a University, but they didn't have a bed, so I had to go to the general psychiatric unit. I mean, very scary. And I was treated with anti-psychotics, antidepressants, and occasional injections to calm me down because I was paranoid, very delusional. **(Margery)**

RESULTS OF UNTREATED PPD

The language used was both physical and directional in nature. Women used directional words, such as through, down, apart, and described the experience in physical terms such as falling, collapse, crumbling, or tumbling. Untreated PPD had a trajectory.

Within a couple of weeks, I totally plummeted to the point that I was emotionally and psychologically pretty catatonic. My husband came home one day and found me sobbing, glazed-eyed on the couch. One kid was in a diaper, nothing else, and I don't know where the other one was. I don't think I'd fed them hardly all day, and everything came tumbling down. **(Dana)**

Having this moment of "I can't go on, and this is all on my shoulders. And if I don't go on, I'm going to die, and my child is going to die." Just this perplexing-crashing-down-on-me emotional place. And that was an energy that carried through that I had to learn to cope with through the postpartum depression. **(Callie)**

Women described a sense of physically breaking apart.

I remember feeling like something cracked open, and I just literally fell to the floor, sobbing. **(Anna)**

For me, it was almost like just breaking. **(Adrienne)**

Basically, it leveled me emotionally and mentally, and physically, and spiritually. **(Paula)**

My whole world was split. **(Haley)**

It just took me to pieces. **(Diana)**

I would say the process was both physically and emotionally shattering. I just felt so raw and open. I was this open wound, and that was the part of the shattering. It cracked me open in a way that everything stung like salt. I felt like I could never heal. **(Helena)**

CONCLUSION

Symptoms speak an important language. For example, a symptom of an underlying bacterial or viral infection is a fever. Until the infection is treated, the fever holds court over the body, making us aware of our illness and signaling to others that we need help. When ignored, the illness turns up the volume on our symptoms; the fever measures our malady.

As we have learned from the women in this book, the symptoms of PPD spoke a similar language. Women knew that something negative was happening, yet due to the lack of preparation in before PPD, they did not know what it was, adding to the distress experienced during PPD.

As we learn in the next chapter, when women sought help for their symptoms of PPD, trusted care providers failed to acknowledge, validate, treat, or refer women to appropriate resources. The distress of the physical and psychological symptoms was exacerbated by the stress of attempting to get help and not receiving it—running the gauntlet to get better, to finally exhale.

CHAPTER 4

RUNNING THE GAUNTLET: PROVIDER FAILURE AND GETTING BETTER

*We hear the words we have spoken, feel our own
blow as we give it, or read in the bystander's eyes the
success or failure of our conduct.*
– William James –

For most women, care providers failed to address PPD, even when women self-disclosed severe symptoms and asked for help. Obstetric/midwifery, general medicine, family medicine, pediatric, mental health, and childbirth professionals were sought out by women for help with symptoms of PPD to no avail. Women's descriptions of care provider failure included inaccurate diagnoses, prescription medication given with no explanation or follow up, referral to providers, who, in turn, failed to return calls, or were unavailable for extended periods, and repeated negligence to ask about symptoms.

The resulting experience was an additional layer of suffering added to the physical and psychological symptoms already occurring and reflected the nature of being unprepared. What follows in part one is a description of how women experienced provider failure by OB/GYN providers, midwives, mental health providers, pediatric providers, lactation consultants, and doulas. Where partners and family members could not provide the clinical assessment and treatment needed, women experienced their darkest hours. Part II describes how these critical moments of desperation lead women to demand treatment, doing whatever it took to end the symptoms and get better.

PART I: THE PROVIDER GAUNTLET

Nobody—my obstetrician, none of my obstetricians had ever mentioned postpartum depression or anything like that to me in any of my prenatal visits, they had never asked me about my own history of any kind of mood or anxiety issues. They never brought it up in any way. **(Georgia)**

Like Georgia, most women reported that care providers failed to address PPD even when women self-disclosed severe symptoms and asked for help.

OB/GYN Provider

Many women experienced provider failure from their OB/GYN, the lack of response to repeated attempts to get care was a significant component of the experience of PPD. Helena told me that after she told her doctor about her symptoms, "The OB was like, 'Oh, you just need to get out and buy a dress.'"

Diana, who experienced suicidal ideation throughout her second pregnancy and after explained,

I tried to talk to my OB about it. I was like, "You know what? I think I'm ready to talk to somebody." And she just said, "Well, I can give you a number for someone. But they're just going to tell you that what you're experiencing is normal." And I was like, well, then screw it, I'm not going to go open my heart out to someone who's going to say, "This is normal." **(Diana)**

Sandy, who took herself to the emergency room after having intrusive thoughts of harming her baby, shared,

> *I was 12 weeks postpartum with my first daughter and made an appointment because I knew things weren't quite right. He told me, "Well, you know you're more than four weeks postpartum, and your hormones should be back to normal by now, and you should be fine. This isn't postpartum depression." He refused to medicate me because I was nursing.* **(Sandy)**

Faith experienced PPD following the births of all three children. With her first baby, Faith said, "I think I went to three different OB/GYNs, and none of them were able to explain what was happening. So, nothing. We just toughed it out." Faith and her husband toughed it out with baby number two as well—assuming there was nothing to be done because the doctor did not know what to do with baby number one. Having suffered twice, when she became pregnant with the third, Faith took special care in choosing a provider. She asked several sources for a referral to someone who would be able to care for her PPD. Faith explained:

> *I had interviewed him before. He was someone that a couple of people in a health system gave credit to for helping some women through postpartum depression. But I completely fell through with him. He did not care for me for the panic and the anxiety. I do feel like he let me down. I ended up under the care of an emergency room physician who quickly prescribed anti-anxiety medication that my own OB had not suggested happening. I don't know what happened, and I don't know whether it was something that was meant to make me stronger. But I certainly fell through the cracks, and it took two and a half years to heal from all of that. So—and I, in turn, became addicted to antianxiety medications.* **(Faith)**

Despite Faith's best efforts to ensure that she would receive appropriate care, yet another OB/GYN failed to provide care. Falling through the cracks resulted in addiction and subsequent rehabilitation.

Midwives

Jamie experienced a home-to-hospital transfer of care for her birth. Her birth team consisted of her midwife, an OB/GYN, labor and delivery nurses, a doula, and a midwifery apprentice. Jamie shared:

> *Nobody on my birth team said anything to me about postpartum depression or birth trauma when it was clear—crystal clear—from the moment my son was born that I needed mental healthcare. I was crying every day with him, all day. I couldn't stop crying. I was constantly upset, and everybody said to me, "Well, you know, if you think you have postpartum depression, then call this number when you get home and everything." And I just remember thinking, are you looking at me? Like, what is wrong with you?* **(Jamie)**

Vicki also experienced an unexpected transfer from homebirth to hospital for the birth of her baby.

> *My midwife was not helpful in any way. She didn't come to the house at all after what happened to me. Once I went into the hospital, I was under an OB's care, and he didn't have any clue about who I was before. My midwife called maybe twice, but she lives in the same town. She lives pretty close. She knew that I was under quite a bit of stress. She called my husband, maybe once, or maybe twice.* **(Vicki)**

Having been failed to be cared for by her midwife, Vicki sought care from a family practitioner, who also failed to address her PPD. Vicki recalled:

I wouldn't send my worst enemy to him now because he didn't help—he should have said, "No, you can't leave this room until you have help." I went to him, like, three times, and he was not supportive in any way. I was like, "Something is physically wrong with me." I thought I was having heart attacks. He just said, "You need to calm down and go to sleep." And it was just so not helpful. It was really bad. I ended up in the ER three times in one week. **(Vicki)**

Grace also had a planned homebirth and eventually ended up at the hospital.

I was in this weird place of having been under the care of midwives, but then also having to have a surgeon for surgery. And even though I was supposed to be under the care of the midwives even postpartum, like, I wasn't getting the care I needed postpartum, and I was in between and calling multiple providers at different offices all the time, like, trying to figure things out, but nobody was really, like, understanding what was going on.

The midwives' office kept saying, like, "You just wait two weeks. You just have to wait two weeks." Like, you know, "It's typical to be sad in the first two weeks." You know? "Just wait two weeks, we can't give you anything for two weeks." I remember thinking, "If this is what is normal, then I don't think anybody would ever have a child. Like, this can't be normal, this feeling that I'm feeling." They were going off the two-week hormone drop. So, they were just saying that I needed to just get to two weeks where my hormones would be more balanced.

The midwives eventually made me a nurse appointment, but they put it under breastfeeding issues, which I really wasn't having, just to get me in. It was with the nurse, not with one of the midwives. I immediately broke down with her and, you know, was visibly upset and kept hearing the two-week thing again. And then she told me a story about a patient that had hid her feelings of suicide from her and eventually told her after she had recovered from her depression and that if I was feeling that way, you know, to give her a call. I just remember thinking, "You're not going to help me. Okay." And just leaving the room, just leaving after that. I stopped calling them after that.

I felt just fully dismissed. Like, it's not bad enough. And so, I just knew that her telling me that, "If you feel like you're going to kill yourself, then that's bad enough to warrant me helping you." She didn't ask me directly if I felt like I was going to hurt myself. She didn't ask me anything about that. I have a medical background, and I think that was another reason why just . . . the way she was interacting with me, I knew that she was, you know, not going to help me.

I felt like I was saying the right thing and just continually being dismissed and being told to wait two weeks and not being provided any other resources. I didn't get any referrals. I contacted the maternal mental health agency here in town myself.

And then I did go to my six-week appointment, and I don't think I was able to really, like, verbalize it what I was going through and had gone through with the midwife. But I filled out the survey form very honestly and took two pages to fill it out and let them know what they had done and what they hadn't done, and it felt so wrong.

I even put my contact information on it. Like, you know, you can leave it private if you want or anonymous if you want. And I chose not to because I was willing to talk about it more. Like, "Be thankful that I wasn't somebody who wanted to take my life." Like, "You could have lost a patient, you know, and that would have been horrible. And also, you could have helped me feel better. And you chose not to." Yeah. But nobody called me.
(Grace)

Similarly, in explaining the care she received for her PPD, Morgan noted the failure of her OB/GYN, and then insufficient treatment by a general practitioner.

> *Well let's see, it wasn't my OB/GYN, it was my general practitioner that kind of knew what I had, but he never really referred to it as postpartum depression. He prescribed me Paxil, and when I asked him why he would put me on an antidepressant if I weren't feeling down. He said, "Well, depression and anxiety, it seems like you have a bit of both. There's a fine line separating the two of them." He knew I was having difficulty sleeping. He knew I was on Ambien. He didn't go into any great detail of why he was prescribing me Paxil over any other antidepressant. Maybe it was successful for most of his patients that experienced something similar to me. And because I was experiencing panic attacks, he put me on Xanax, which I was on for a couple of weeks. Somehow, I survived.* **(Morgan)**

Mental Health Providers

In addition to obstetrics, midwifery, family, and general medical care providers, mental health providers also failed to help. Misdiagnosis was a prominent experience for Deborah, who had been given a diagnosis of bipolar disorder one year prior to her pregnancy by a reputable psychiatrist. I went to this psychiatrist at a local university medical center. They have a whole clinic for women who are pregnant or wan. They're experts in, like, the pharmaceutical part of it.

> *But no, she actually misdiagnosed me years before as on the bipolar spectrum because I had had what I now know what as a long panic episode, and she thought it was hypomanic, and she was wrong. But for whatever reason, she was not willing to*

rethink her diagnosis or my treatment plan. So, I just got the wrong treatment for a very long time.

But I, you know, I believed her. And she was not trained in CBT. She was a very traditional talk therapist. Like, there was no strategy, it was just talk therapy, which at one point in my life was fine, and then all of a sudden was not. So, I made the change; it took me a long time to figure out and to kind of get the balls to get someone new, and finding someone new can be overwhelming when you've been in the care of someone else for so long.

So, my current clinician was looking through my records, and she said, "I don't see an anxiety diagnosis." I'm like, "There isn't one." And she also was like, "I'm sorry, what?" Needless to say, there was a lot of anger and frustration on my part, and a lot of, like, "Why didn't you see this sooner? You are not stupid, and you know, you've been in various kinds of therapy for most of your post-adolescent life." You know, why didn't I make a change earlier? And so, what I've tried to come to accept that my other provider should have realized what was going on and should have send me to someone who does CBT. **(Deborah)**

Janis told me:

I ended up going to—needing urgent care because I couldn't get into psychiatry for treatment. I started working with a therapist, started seeing a therapist, and then was waiting to get some medication. So, I was waiting to see the psychiatrist. Every single moment felt so incredibly painful and frightening. I ended up going to the emergency room for help. I felt more vulnerable than I ever have. **(Janis)**

Beatrice shared how her experience with a psychologist resulted in her not getting the care she needed.

The professional help I did try, the lady was honestly very, very rude to me on the phone. We kept playing phone tag, and finally,

when I got a hold of her, she said to me, "Like, what do you want?"
Like, very meanly and rudely, and I was just so taken aback, espe-
cially since I had training as a therapist. It was so inappropriate.
I had explained to her what I was going through, and she said,
"Well, I'm too far for you to drive," and she didn't have anyone—
any other name to give me. So, I just didn't reach out for help
after that. **(Beatrice)**

Diana, who ended up suicidal and hospitalized, reported similar
provider failure when she sought help from a psychiatrist.

I tried to go to a psychiatrist, and they told me to turn on my iPod
when my baby cried, and then I went to a therapist, and she's like,
"I don't know what's going on." And she said, "Do you think you're
the only mother to ever experience anxiety?" **(Diana)**

Helena also experienced provider failure from a mental health
professional who dismissed her with inappropriate feedback;
"They said, 'Oh, it sounds like you and your husband are really
struggling, and let's focus on the marriage.'"

In a stunning experience of psychiatric provider failure, Callie
describes her first attempt at in-treatment care.

So, I decided to go to this treatment facility in New Mexico,
which is supposed to be the best in mind, body, spirit. Who I
was then, it's like, "So, I'm going to do it all the way. And I'm
going to fix myself and I . . ." You know, that was a different
part of my personality that needed to be healed and seen. I can
laugh at it now. And I have those aspects still, but you know.
So, I went away for six weeks to get treatments. And this ho-
listic facility, I'll say, on the one hand, I did breathwork when
I was there.

And that was a wonderful experience because unbeknownst to me,
I'm doing breathwork, and all of a sudden, all of this scream came

out of me that I had held on to when I was in the hospital birthing my son because I didn't want to yell. And it was very healing to just touched upon through breathwork and experience that. And I think that's the only good thing about that facility because they took me off of all my medications and I was completely unstable.

And it was very, in my opinion, the treatment out there, there's so much mental health stigma, even practitioners who are in the field, and it was just not good. But luckily, I left there within ten days, and I found another treatment facility, and they put me on more powerful medication that ended up stabilizing me. And then, you know, until you're stable, you can't really, you know, do your work. And I didn't need to be flooded. I was already flooded. I didn't need to be doing breathwork and EMDR, and I found another facility shortly after. **(Callie)**

Pediatric Care Providers

Other postpartum care providers were sought out for help and failed to acknowledge, address, or provide care, even when asked. For example, remember that Sandy ended up with thoughts of harming her daughter due to a lack of treatment. She had sought support from her daughter's pediatrician, and recalled:

I remember talking to my daughter's pediatrician. We actually begged him for a night nurse for her, and he was like, "Why do you need one?" I'm like, "I'm not doing well because she needs to be fed around the clock. We're exhausted. He has to work. And I'm pumping 24/7, and we need someone." And he's like, "Well, your insurance and Medicaid won't cover it." And he refused to, and he, like, practically laughed at us about it. I'm, like, I need this help and you're just laughing about it? **(Sandy)**

For Anna, who was having thoughts of driving her car into oncoming traffic, it was a visiting nurse who failed to provide much-needed care.

Here is this visiting nurse here to help [the baby]. She goes through the checklist, and she says, "Oh, are you having any postpartum depression thoughts? Oh well, clearly, you're not having a problem with that." And she literally checked her box off and moved on. **(Anna)**

Lactation Consultants

For Betsy, problems with breastfeeding resulted in attentive care from lactation nurses and lactation consultants. However, the care provided was for breastfeeding and failed to address Betsy's PPD symptoms.

No one, even though I had been like to all these nurses and lactation consultants trying to breastfeed, no one had—they all just stared at my chest and my baby. Nobody actually talked to me and asked how I was doing. I remember we had this one lactation consultant who, actually, I really liked, who came in for like the whole day to be with us. She's like a crazy-lactation-consultant-to-the-stars woman. And I haven't seen the video, but I've seen the photos, still photos from that day, and I looked so bad. There's no way anyone in their right mind could look at me and think that I was okay. Because I've seen enough women postpartum now to know, you know, obviously no one looks great physically, but you know. You're tired.

I know how I looked the second time around, and I'm sure I looked tired, but I also was happy and could smile and could—like, my eyes didn't have that glazed overlook, you know. And I remember her being really sweet and nice about—and telling me, in terms of the breastfeeding issues. And making me feel like that was okay and being very comforting. But she never asked—you know, she asked me everything about how I was feeling and his birth. Why didn't she ever just look into my eyes and say, "How are you?" **(Betsy)**

Deborah also described how lactation consultants failed to treat her, appropriately.

I think I probably got better care than a lot of women did, but in particular, finding out that they piece around nursing was so unfairly blamed on me when it was a physical issue. It was a biological issue. I think that mourning the loss of nursing for me was actually a really big part of how quickly I got depressed. So, if any one person had said to me at the hospital, "You know what? This may not be your fault."

I was trying to pump around the clock with a baby that wouldn't sleep, and it was just . . . that was awful. I think I probably got better care than a lot of women did, but in particular, finding out that they piece around nursing was so unfairly blamed on me when it was a physical issue; it was a biological issue.

I switched OBs after my son was born. The OB I'm currently with is much more versed in PCOS. When I described to her the lack of lactation after his birth, she said, "Well, that's a known PCOS complication." I said, "Excuse me?" She was like, "You never had a provider tell you that? You never had a provider tell you that this may be totally physiological and not something you can help?" I said, "Not one. Not one person."

No one had told me about PCOS and lactation issues. Not my therapist, not my OB, not the lactation consultant, not the nurses, nobody. All they kept telling me was, "Drink this tea, eat these oats. Drink a Guinness. Pump, pump, pump. Just keep putting him on your boob, just keep putting him on your boob." It was crazy making at the time. That was almost a bigger trauma than anything else. **(Deborah)**

Doulas

As previously noted, part of Jamie's birth team included a birth doula. Birth doulas are trained to provide emotional support to the laboring woman during her birth and provide resources and support for a woman in the immediate postpartum period. For Jamie, her doula was yet another source of provider failure, not only due to not screening, for failing to acknowledge what she experienced as immediate and apparent mental distress.

> *My doula never said anything to me about it. But when I went to that therapist postpartum, there was a day when I went with my son because I couldn't get a babysitter and guess who came out before me? My doula. I was about four months postpartum, and she was about two, and she was with her baby and crying. Later, I sent her an e-mail, and I said, "I don't want to be nosey, but I saw you in a psychiatrist waiting room, and we hugged, and I hope that wasn't awkward. I didn't want to violate your boundaries. I just hope that you're okay." She said, "Oh, this is the second time I've had postpartum depression." And I thought, why didn't you share your story with me? That would have been great, you know.* **(Jamie)**

Partners and Family

In addition to care providers failing to acknowledge and respond to women's symptoms, some women reported that their partners or family members failed to provide care despite their obvious signs of PPD. Mindy shared an experience with her husband.

> *Even though I told him I had a postpartum mood disorder, he just dismissed me. And then when I started working on my photography project about PPD, he was dismissive of that until he actually heard some of the audio of women speaking about*

their PPD. Then I think it started bringing out fear in him. A few times, he actually said, "Do I need to take the kids from you?" That was how he responded to all of this. As opposed to listening, it was all fear-based. (**Mindy**)

Similarly, Skye described her husband's failure to address her worsening symptoms.

He left and went to work. Here I was, sick, with this newborn sitting next to me, and I totally felt abandoned, and overwhelmed, and sick, and it was awful. I mean, it was terrible. And I know my husband's a good man, but he was just feeling overwhelmed with the pressure of "I have to make this money for us and stuff." So, I don't really blame him, but it's hard not to sometimes. It's, like, really? I was totally sick. But I don't even think he was around enough to really realize how sick I was or how bad it was. (**Skye**)

Darkest Hours

The heartbreak and frustration described did not occur in isolation from the experience and demands of motherhood. Women experienced debilitating physical and emotional symptoms of PPD while simultaneously engaged in caring for their newborn, including breastfeeding, physical recovery from childbirth (including wound care), and returning to normal daily functions of work inside and outside of the home. In some cases, women were caring for multiple children or had additional stressors of an out of state move, postpartum uterine infection, difficulty breastfeeding, or mastitis.

The consequence of the multiple obstacles to treatment was a worsening of symptoms as demands to care for a newborn and return to daily functioning increased. Navigating the maze of the healthcare system and persevering through provider failure to recognize or treat PPD created a dangerous progression of symptoms. Several women expressed a series of failures from multiple providers, contributing to an experience of hopelessness, distress, and confusion, as Helena described.

> *Part of my frustration was with trying to navigate the healthcare system because I was trying to reach out—I thought, maybe, these might be exit doors or ladders to get out of the maze or something. And I just kept having one door after another shut on me. It was like, who will listen to me? That's why I had to keep running this gauntlet because nobody was seeing it, only I was, and it was very lonely. There were a lot of dark hours because it seemed like every time I tried, again, another door shut in my face. I did keep trying, but a lot of women don't.* **(Helena)**

As I analyzed these data, images of the walking wounded came to mind, as if these women were hemorrhaging blood—in public—and no one noticed. The experience of being symptomatic and yet invisible to providers was a profound feeling of utter despair in flesh and form. To walk through daily life dying and being ignored by care providers, and invisible to support systems was crazy-making and cruel.

There was almost a punitive sense of the experience of care provider failure: an additional layer of humiliation, indignity, and negligence. The lack of reaction from providers was an insult on top of the injury. On some level, the systemic lack of treatment created the causes for the growth of powerful resilience and determination. In other words, women got pragmatic. If their providers were not going to fix the problem, they would do it themselves, as Jamie described,

> *No one can do this but me. I have to figure out a way to get through this. And that's when I realized "okay, you have to*

work. You have to figure this out." That was the moment I started getting better. **(Jamie)**

Turning Points in Transformation

In her 2013 book *Stay,* poet and philosopher Jennifer Michael Hecht chronicled the history of suicide as a plea to readers to "choose to stay" (p. 234). Choosing to heal is hard work. Deciding not to attempt suicide is hard work. It requires heavy lifting.

The heavy lifting of healing noted in this chapter include women disclosing the gravity of their symptoms to others, not knowing what the response might bring. In any case, women did it. They faced unknown outcomes of disclosing their illness and braced for the fall-out—determined to do what it took to get better. Paula, who had been plagued by intrusive thoughts of suicidal ideation, told me how she had reached a turning point when she disclosed to a family member.

> *I knew I couldn't keep going like that. So, I called a cousin of mine who is a social worker and told her, "I need to be seen right away. I need you to help me." She was my lifeline—I finally said out loud for the first time, "I think I'm suffering from postpartum depression." As soon as I got the sentence out, I burst into tears. I knew that I was—if I didn't get help, I was going to be in a crisis at some point, and I didn't want to take that chance.* **(Paula)**

Paula told me that then she asked her cousin to write down exactly what to say, "so that I would be seen right away, but so they wouldn't think that I was a danger to myself or my children."

Jamie shared how she finally admitted the extent of her symptoms during a phone conversation with her therapist.

I told her, "I just can't do this anymore. I feel like I've fallen through a hole in space and time, and I feel like somewhere, there's the real me, living my old life where I don't have a baby, and I'm happy, and I'm confident, and I'm like I used to be. I'm in this universe that's all wrong, where everything's just wrong. And I'm not supposed to be a mother, and this was a big mistake. You know, my husband will meet someone else. His mother will take care of the baby. I just don't want to be here anymore. I just don't want to do this, and I don't think that I'm doing my son any good."

She had this answer for me that just like zapped me: "You know, I've treated people in my practice whose parents killed themselves and you need to know that your son will never be okay. And your husband, he will never be okay. Nobody is ever going to be okay. Your son doesn't need a mother; he needs you. You are the one."

When she said that, I just was suddenly like, "Oh my God, like I have to do this work, there's no other choice." I remember crying a lot, and I just told her, "Okay, I'll do the work. I'll do whatever it takes, but you have to help me because I don't know what to do." **(Jamie)**

PART II: GETTING BETTER BY ENDING THE SYMPTOMS

Given the severity of symptoms, the lack of information, and the gauntlet women had to run in order to access treatment—how did they get better? I asked the question—What were the ways you saw yourself transforming?—to probe for specific patterns related to how women transitioned from shattered to transformed. For every woman, stopping the symptoms was a turning point in the process of transformation.

As noted, disclosing to providers that they were sick didn't end the symptoms. They were either not treated or told they had to wait nearly two months for treatment. Those who were given treatment were either given the wrong treatment, such as the wrong medication, or the wrong diagnosis. Emergency room doctors, rather than specialists, treated many others.

Women knew that they were receiving random, if not haphazard, prescribed medications. They heard the condescending suggestions of buying a new dress or turning on the iPod when the baby cried. At the intersection of the most severe suffering and recovery, women knew they were being given bad treatment, no treatment, or insulting anecdotes. The infantilizing of their experience did not go unnoticed. However, women weathered the worst in order to end the symptoms.

Diana told me stories of the ridiculous group activity exercises she was asked to do during her hospitalization for suicidal ideation due to untreated PPD. Yet, she still found being admitted helpful. She shared how she would pull a particular nurse's aside for advice and conversation, and just endured the sing-along music therapy. For Diana, "Inpatient was helpful in that I got a break, and I got to get away, and I got a couple good pieces of advice."

Sienna, who spent a month having her husband hide her medication every night so that she wouldn't overdose, told me how uncomfortable group exercises at outpatient treatment were for her. *"We had to go every day and talk about how suicidal we were and how we were feeling that day."* But then she explained that she had been so sick from her depression, it was worth it. *"I was so desperately seeking a cure, seeking to get over it, I reached out to every avenue and did everything possible."* **(Sienna)**

Grace's description and the nature of the wording speaks to the "if I don't do something" nature of getting better.

I think my biggest thing was that I just, like, the thought. I mean, when you're going through an anxiety attack or going through depression, your thoughts tell you to like, "This is never going to end," right? And just having that feeling of, like, "I can't. I can't live like this," like, this is, like, "I can't do this." Like, I have to try everything to make this go away." I was willing to take any medication that they would give me. I just wanted the feelings to stop, you know. So, I think that's what really guided me is just that intense urge just to make it stop. **(Grace)**

Ending the symptoms of PPD meant enduring indignities and embarrassment. Still, regardless of the quality of care, women made choices that they wouldn't otherwise make, in order to just have the symptoms end. There was a relationship between the severity of illness and willingness to try anything to make it better. There was a relationship between women being ignored in systems of power and rising to take care of themselves despite all odds, or recommendations. And there was a relationship between the experience of PPD and experience of an exposure to life-threatening events, as in a traumatic event.

Haley, who had "lived with depression for a while before ever seeking help for it" became proactive in her care, telling her therapist that she needed specific help.

I just kept soldiering on and marching through it. It wasn't until I took the time to kind of really listen to my body and myself that I realized that I needed help. So, I called, and within, I want to say, like, two days of my first phone call, I was meeting with my therapist, and a couple of weeks later, I was started on medication. **(Haley)**

Haley did the work of getting better herself. She called the therapist; she waited "a couple of weeks" to get treated, which also meant enduring those weeks while still ill from depression and taking care of a newborn. She then handled taking psychotropic medication for the first time in her life, while trying to understand side effects, how and when to take the medication, and waiting for them to actually work (psychotropic medication can take up to four weeks to metabolize and address symptoms).

Haley's experience reminded me of someone with a debilitating migraine headache, having to call the doctor, wait two weeks for an appointment while still having the headache, and taking care of a baby. Then, taking the medication and putting up with negative side effects for a month before the headache starts to subside. Can you imagine?

Doing Whatever it Took

With no follow-up care provided after the emergency department doctor prescribed powerful anti-anxiety medication, Faith told me that she had to get treatment for dependency on anti-anxiety medication. A soft-spoken mother of three with no prior history of substance abuse, Faith described, *"I would do it all over again. I would do the panic and the anxiety medication again because I don't think I'd be here today if I hadn't."* Faith knew that she would have attempted suicide if she hadn't gotten herself to the emergency room. And while becoming addicted to anti-anxiety medication was a horrible side effect, in hindsight, Faith knew it saved her life.

For Beatrice, her experience of getting help hinged on a close relationship with a friend across the country. As Beatrice came to describe this friend during our interview, she began to cry—almost suddenly. The tears took her off guard, as we had been talking for nearly an hour and she hadn't been tearful. When she mentioned her friend, she recalled how her friend saved her life.

My friend said to me, "You have postpartum depression." I was like, "Well, there's nothing I can do about it. I'm in trouble, but there's nothing I can do." My friend was on a message board with someone in Miami, near me. She emailed her and said, "Please, help my friend. Please, help her." And when that woman reached out to me, that was the beginning of getting better. **(Beatrice)**

Education

Following Margery's experience, she sought further psychoeducation as a lifeline to recovery.

I felt like recovery was on my own. But I did everything I could to do classes and learn about behavioral and mental health at the local behavioral health center. They have classes every day from, like, 9 to 12. And I'd go and learn. I mean, nurses are always learning, and that was just the beginning of a way for me to dig into more knowledge and my own treatment plan. Because what they were giving me wasn't enough. **(Margery)**

Other Providers: Lifelines

For two women, their babies' pediatrician served as a lifeline. Betsy described:

I remember at my son's, I think, 2-week appointment, and I still, to this day, I credit her with saving me. She was so amazing. I remember she finished the appointment, and she just turned to me and said, "How are you doing, Mom?" And it was the first someone had asked me that. She said it so matter-of-factly. I was, like, okay, I need to tell somebody. That was the first time I voiced it, but I remember saying very clearly, "I think I have postpartum depression," to anyone. **(Betsy)**

Mindy said,

Postpartum depression was not in the forefront of my mind (or anyone else for that matter) until I spoke to my daughter's pediatrician.

I had been into the office a few times, and this doctor saw something in me that I wasn't seeing in myself. A floodgate opened because she shared with me everything I'd been feeling, and I pushed it away. I thought I was a horrible mom. I couldn't understand the thoughts I was having. To have someone say those things out loud, and in a way that I didn't feel ashamed, was so empowering. **(Mindy)**

For Mindy, accessing complementary and alternative medicine (CAM) was a key component to her getting better. Again, Mindy sought out this care herself. Finally, getting better for Mindy also involved getting out of the house and getting behind a camera.

I sought out acupuncture, and my acupuncturist also does some therapy with it, and she had experience dealing with women who had postpartum depression. I was extremely, extremely anemic. We did blood work. We talked about St. John's wort. We talked antidepressants.

After I started getting treatment, I started recognizing when I had to get out of the house. I was a stay-at-home mom, and all these thoughts and stuff were—a lot of the things were fear-based. So, I never wanted to leave the house. I never wanted to leave the kids. I had all sorts of fears. When I finally started getting treatment, and kind of had a little bit more clear thinking, I recognized the fact that I needed to get out and do something.

When my son was born, I picked up a camera just to kind of keep my creative flow going, and even while I was going through this, I'd bring out my camera because if I would get really anxious or really depressed, or angry, or anything when Lucy was around, I decided to take photos. **(Mindy)**

Mindy explained that the experience of getting behind the lens provided a sense of cover for her symptoms while serving her desire to attend to and care for her children. Many struggled with the perception that their babies and children would suffer if they saw their affect. In other words, women were greatly concerned that their visual presentation of symptoms would negatively affect their babies.

This concern was mediated for Mindy by using a camera. The lens of a camera made Mindy feel that she was simultaneously shielding her children from seeing her hurting while providing her a vehicle to express her awe-inspiring love of as a mother. Using a camera might be a novel intervention for women suffering from PPD to be explored in future research.

For Callie, her therapist was her "anchor."

I saw her twice a week. If in between, I was having a crisis, I would call her on the phone, 20 minutes, boom, it was like . . . you know, I've always been an athlete, I was a rugby player for 10 years. You know, anything I put my mind to, I could do. This was entirely different. But that energy and that ability, it was like she was my coach. "Okay, here's what we're going to do to me next." "Okay, I can do it." You know, because it's just terrifying, absolutely terrifying.

And for me, mindfulness, my spirituality is a huge component because I could see. At least I could see. I knew where I was. And like my therapist says, "I've never seen someone worked so hard to get out of that place." I was not staying there. No way. No how. It was just what I'm describing, terrifying. **(Callie)**

Adrienne's lifeline was her lactation consultant:

My lactation consultant, finally, after I was released from the psychiatric facility in the hospital, took me up to her office to pump because it had been quite a long time, and I needed to come. And she said, "So what medications do they have you on?" And I said, "Zoloft, and they gave me Ambien, but I still can't sleep." And she said, "Oh, that's because of anxiety and not . . . You don't need an Ambien for that. That won't work." So, she advocated again on my behalf and called my doctor, and got me the script for Ativan so that I could keep breastfeeding because it's short-acting, no negative effects in terms of fractional, so I can keep going but also sleep.

Once I got into a regular pattern of sleeping a bit more, the medications took hold in that four to six weeks. It probably took a good- I want to say one to two months. I remember the day I went into the hospital was in August. I think I really started feeling much better in the beginning of October. I do have a memory of being able to go out trick-or-treating with my kids, and actually enjoy it, and want to do it, and want to be able to step out of the house and go places, and actually spend time with my family and my children. **(Adrienne)**

Support Groups

Many women described the role of support groups as a critical component of getting better. It is important to reiterate that while the support group was a community that helped to heal, it took individual initiative to find the group, attend the group, and keep going to the group. In the middle of a crisis, women used extraordinary strength to get support. Support groups don't just appear in your living room—it takes work to find them and physically go to the meeting while juggling infant care, breastfeeding, and the physical symptoms of an illness that include extreme exhaustion. Still, they persisted. Anna said,

I really felt the switch flip when I started talk therapy and medication, and within probably, two or three weeks of that, I started in our postpartum support group. That was very powerful. I just let myself be very open with women who I had never met before. I distinctly remember crying pretty much throughout the entire meeting. But freeing myself to be so open with strangers about something that I couldn't clearly articulate to even my closest friends or family was a big breakthrough for me. It was a blessing to have a group of people who had been through the same thing and who were describing the same things—you could swear they were reading your mind! **(Anna)**

Adrienne adds,

I ended up calling Postpartum Support International and their warm line and actually got through to someone, and she, by heaven hand, picked up the phone and answered my call. And right away, she was able to empathize with me to validate how I was feeling and, you know, offered me information about who I can see and reach out to psychiatrists, psychologists. **(Adrienne)**

Combined Methods of Recovery

For many, like Callie, finding the right combination of treatments included trying multiple modalities.

I remember, white-knuckling, and driving down the road and having those intrusive thoughts. Truly, like I explained it, and that's why, to this day, I'm on medication. And I really, truly thought when I got off, when I started to heal from postpartum depression because I was on a concoction. I had an antidepressant, lithium, and antipsychotics.

So, I had that right combination that gave me that stability at the time. And then as I became well and whole and started taking those steps, I got right off the antidepressant, I got right off the lithium. And then I was going to get off the last one, the antipsychotic, and everything, whoa. I thought I had that internalized stigma where I truly thought, like, getting off medication means I'm cured. I'm well. And I didn't realize the stigma that I had.

And I don't relate to it now because the last medication, the antipsychotic, I need that. I have no problem taking that. And I thank God that we have medications.

Then I did electric shock therapy at my . . . it was the next step. I would say that that was positive. That was the first time in proba-bly . . . you know, because that was about almost ten months into it. And I will tell you what I do remember is coming out from one of those treatments, and it felt like, karmically, I had been underwater and I, for the first time, came up and was gasping for air. And I, at that moment, remembered how much I loved my husband and my children, for the first time. And if that was the only thing I got from it, that was enough. And it was after that that I got—found the right psychiatrist. And then I got the stability I needed. And it was after that I started taking steps. **(Callie)**

Karen explained how a combination of support systems, medication, spirituality, and therapy worked in concert to help her.

So, the first thing was the level of support that my family was able to give me. Second, I'm Catholic, so I believe in God, and I believe that He gave me a gift in that [my daughter] has nothing wrong with her . . . And so, all of those things together, and my husband is really supportive. He has been nothing but supportive. And I took medication. The other big piece is that taking medication, which is, I think, the accepting help too. **(Karen)**

Women reflected on an overwhelming sense of gratitude to the specific individual or groups who facilitated getting symptoms addressed. Women explained that finally having their suffering acknowledged was a turning point in their recovery and trans-formation, and many referred to this experience as a lifeline. Lifelines were in the form of resources not previously tapped: friends, rel-atives, therapists, pediatricians, and support groups.

CONCLUSION

Getting better was both an end of the symptoms and a shifted worldview toward new possibilities. A critical component of the shift to recovery and beyond was the experience of being seen, heard, and accepted. The range of this experience was broad, but the underlying theme was becoming visible. Finally having someone acknowledge that they had PPD resulted in a release of potential life changes never considered before.

CHAPTER 5

AFTER POSTPARTUM DEPRESSION: I AM A DIFFERENT PERSON

I don't want to make somebody else.
I want to make myself.
– Toni Morrison, *Sula* –

From a general outlook to specific observations, women described the process of transformation by explaining the ways they saw themselves changed by PPD. They saw changes in their sense of self, relationships, and their role in the world was noted.

I was struck by how clearly women knew their answers. There was no hesitation in their speech, no searching for words, no pauses. Here, the energy of the interviews developed momentum, and women cited examples of how they experienced themselves as transformed with excitement and clarity.

So, it's definitely transformed my view of the world, and my view of my life, and my view that I own my life; my life doesn't own me. **(Diana)**

In a broader sense, my overall attitude and outlook on life is just a lot more positive. When things go wrong, I can generally laugh about it now or be humorously sarcastic about it as opposed to, "oh, this is more evidence that the sky is falling, Chicken Little kind of thing." I was just more willing to explore that kind of thinking and come out on the other side of exploring that feeling positive and encouraged.

So yeah, I think there was definitely a big shift just in my overall approach to small details and broader concepts of how you live life. (**Dana**)

PART 1: TRANSFORMED SENSE OF SELF

A significant component of the paradigm shift described after PPD was observed in changed beliefs, behaviors, and attitudes regarding self-care. Anna described new behaviors and values regarding increased self-awareness.

I feel like my experience with postpartum depression and recovering from postpartum depression really illustrated the importance of self-awareness. I think that the most marked part of the transformation for me is that I feel like I work harder to be attuned to what I need and kind of checking in with myself to know how I'm feeling and what I need. Whether it's to recharge myself or to have a physical outlet of exercise or sleep, or an emotional need for connecting with someone or being able to vent or communicate how I'm feeling about something. I don't know that I allowed myself the time and space to do those things before that experience. (**Anna**)

Self-Care: Self-Advocacy

For some, changes in self-care involved changing how they communicated to others and eliminating negative self-talk. In our interview, Paula mentioned several times that she took a "long, hard look" at her negative self-talk postpartum, making a conscious effort to focus on positive aspects of herself after PPD. Jamie also described that after PPD, she changed her self-talk.

I've learned to talk to myself the way I would want my son spoken to—with kindness. I've become a lot kinder to myself because I've

figured out that self-kindness is the only way out of those dark places.
(Jamie)

Several women discussed developing a transformed sense of self-kindness and self-advocacy after recovering from untreated PPD. Grace reflected on her newfound ability to advocate for her thyroid condition in this way.

I used to push down my voice and what I needed, and never really letting that out. Whereas now, I speak about it much more freely and say what I need. For example, I need to draw a boundary around what we're doing this weekend because I have only so much energy. It has to be from me. I have to be able to take care of myself but also decide myself that that's what I want to do with my very precious time on this earth like everyone does.

I think that finding my voice and my power was amplified completely through my experience of postpartum depression and anxiety. I really think that was, like a switch in the way, and I am able to advocate more for myself, put boundaries in place for myself, and advocate for others. **(Grace)**

Sandy used similar language:

Postpartum depression really taught me how to take care of myself and be kind to myself. I always enjoyed doing things that made me happy, but now it's, like, okay, I have to do this. This is part of what I have to do to survive. Going through postpartum created a lot of positive behaviors that I have incorporated into life now, and I'm actually grateful for it. So, it's a huge growth process, but for me, it was really looking at myself and trying to figure out who I had become, who I wanted to be, and how much time I was willing to take for myself on the whole motherhood process. **(Sandy)**

After getting treated and recovering from PPD, women prioritized their own needs more seriously than before.

I've learned to listen to myself a lot more, be a little more "selfish" about what I need. Where before, it was more outward, making sure everyone else had what they had. **(Haley)**

My prioritizing myself. I'm allowing myself to do that. It's something I have to do multiple times a day is reminding myself to prioritize me. **(Janis)**

I have the realization that I deserve to exist. And so that kind of realization also means I deserve to have certain things. I've given myself the space to go slow, which is hard for me. I like to just get things done and do it. Now I give myself more time. Less pressure on myself. **(Karen)**

Going slowly, listening to internal cues, and prioritizing one's needs and value distinguished the description of self- care for women reflected in the text. Transformed self-care behaviors were incorporated into daily life and accompanied by a new sense of confidence, living authentically, and being honest and open about PPD and motherhood. As Karen noted, a new sense of self-worth contributed to positive growth and sustained recovery. The assumptive world was being rebuilt.

Confidence

Out of 25 interviews, 21 women used the phrase, "If I can live through that, I can live through anything"—an emblematic statement of the realization of self-determination and strength in the face of extreme challenge. Women explained a new sense of confidence, a sense of hard-won wisdom:

I felt like I had been through the worst at the beginning and lived to tell the tale, so, you know, no matter what I faced from then on, I then had the tools to handle it because I had done the work and gotten through that, that initial hell. (**Betsy**)

So, it feels like I've been to hell and back, you know. I can take on people. I mean, I'm just not scared of things that I used to be scared of. (**Sienna**)

It's almost like I want to say, "Don't mess with me, I have been through hell and back again, and I will knock you down just to protect this person." (**Faith**)

So, through this experience, I'm actually becoming a much stronger woman in my own life, and I'm continuing to move forward in that way. (**Mindy**)

I have more confidence in myself and my ability to make decisions. I'm okay. It's definitely helped me become more confident and more self-aware of who I am and what I need. I trust myself where before I wasn't. I was always doubting myself. So, I'm proud of myself and, you know, saying I'm confident in who I am, for the most part, is huge. (**Haley**)

I just feel so empowered and so strong as a person for coming through PPD. I just know that if I can get through that, and feel the way I feel now, I can do anything. I feel like a superwoman most of the time. (**Diana**)

Women also reported a willingness to try new activities, new communication styles at work, and in relationships and approaching new relationships:

I'm much more willing to go out and just explore and live, I guess, and actually, you know, do things instead of just, like, I don't know if I should, and I'm not as intimidated anymore. **(Sandy)**

I approached someone that I admired her writing, and I knew she was a local writer to me, and I said, "Would you like to come out for coffee?" And now, she and I are part of this collaboration where we're bringing storytelling experience to our city, and that would have never happened before because I would have been too afraid to be bold and to take risks. **(Paula)**

And also, like trying new things-- I got really into yoga and Bikram. And I started that about two months ago. I started it because one I thought it would be good for the mind and body. I never would have even tried or thought about doing yoga in a hot room, but it was kind of like, "Go big or go home!" I felt empowered to do it. I needed to sweat out all these bad feelings and center myself. **(Sienna)**

Sienna went on to express that her behavior at work had changed, and that her overall appreciation for life had been transformed.

I've become more empowered in all areas of my life. Things I was once afraid of, I'm not as afraid now. I'm more assertive at work, a little bit. I mean, I've always kind of been passive-aggressive. Now I'm not, you know, aggressive in any means, but I'm just more confident because I know that I got through that. **(Sienna)**

Reflections on the development of new strengths included the new capacity for caring for themselves and for others. Integrating honest, authentic perceptions of the difficulties of motherhood co-occurred with the experience of being less judgmental, more compassionate, and more confident to try new things and establish new relationships.

Authenticity

The ways women saw themselves transforming included an increased sense of personal authenticity, honesty regarding PPD, and a sense of being real about the difficulty of motherhood.

> It's almost like the whole experience caused me to look inward and reevaluate in a lot of ways. **(Betsy)**

> It's almost like the postpartum depression was a gift because it gave, like, a cover under, which I could go and seek help. Little did I know, I was seeking help for something that I had been dealing with all of my adult life for sure, and probably a good stretch of my entire life. In addition to my own healing and finding just what I really feel like is just a better, more authentic way to live my life. I also, what the experience also gave me is, like, I don't need the cover anymore. **(Georgia)**

> I grew up in a situation where I had an adopted older brother who would be considered a conduct disorder. He would be considered an antisocial personality. And he abused me for 18 years, sexually. So, I have quite the story. And yet, I don't identify with that anymore. But back then, during PPD, that was the part of me that was trapped in silence. That vulnerable person who was ashamed and couldn't speak and couldn't share her truth and couldn't be seen.

> I explained this to my son. There's a difference between fitting in and belonging. You know, fitting in is going out into your environment, and you're analyzing it and your interpreting it, and you're like, "This is what I have to do to fit in." But belonging is

the opposite. It is knowing who you are and it's taking the risk and the courage to share vulnerably who you are and to be brave enough to set boundaries and let go of people that don't serve you and being very clear about who you are and who you're not. And finding a place where you're, like, "This is where I belong. This is who I am." So, I discovered that in the process too. I mean, there's so many aspects of this whole process and journey. **(Callie)**

I'm very open about it. I don't think I had a choice, really. I think mine was so severe that there was no hiding it. I want to spread awareness about it. I think a lot of people think that postpartum depression is equal to postpartum psychosis in that the mother kills her babies or does something, you know, kills herself. I think people get it confused. I've been open about it on Facebook, even to my over 500 friends through past college friends and everything, because I want to spread awareness, and I want to help any other mom that's going through it. I feel like I can just be truthful with people and be honest with people, and I'm not really as worried about what they think. **(Sienna)**

I'm brutally honest. I don't mince words about how I feel about something. That said, I do try to be tactful about it, but I'm like, "No, I'm not comfortable with this, so no, I'm not going to do it, and it's okay that I don't want to do it." **(Sandy)**

My coworker's spouse took her child's life. She was suffering from postpartum psychosis. You know it's not often that you have a team meeting, and they talk about what had happened because it was in the news, and he's like, "Do you have any questions?" And I just started crying in front of the entire team, and I said, "This is why this is important to me. This is why it's upsetting to me personally."

We're just a small team of four, and one woman had a daughter, and she never went through it, and neither did her daughter, so she really just wanted to understand. So, I just really talked about this is what it's like, explained all the different mood disorders; here's my struggles, this is what I did to get better. Then with the coworker, with the spouse, the same thing. I just really said, "I feel for her because here's someone in our own midst that had he'd known that I'd suffered and I blog now, and I'm telling my story, and gosh, I wish I knew because there are so many resources I could have given him and given to his wife." It also made me realize what a great team I had because, really, the team came in support of my coworker—and my boss was really understanding. (Paula)

Honesty about Motherhood

Increased authenticity as an awareness of needing honesty regarding the demands of motherhood was described. One of my favorite statements came from Diana, who said, "I don't know why we won't tell each other it sucks, man." This awareness was echoed by many.

I mean, I put so much stress on myself to try and be this picture-perfect mom, and I've realized through this experience and through all these things, that I just need to be who I am and if I am happy with who I am and comfortable, and confident that's going to be the most important things for my kids. Not whether or not I'm the craftiest mom, and I'm going to hand sew all their clothes, hand-knit everything, and be this incredible baker and cook. I mean, I had this idealistic picture. **(Mindy)**

New, realistic interpretations of motherhood replaced previously held unrealistic standards of perfection. A component of transformation involved increased authenticity regarding being a "good mom," as Karen explained:

I've realized what I kind of need as a person, and that realization of okay, these are some of the pieces of what I need to be a good mom. Things like I need to work. I need to go outside of raising my daughter. I tried staying home for a while afterward because it was so intense. So, realizing that and being okay with that, I think, was hard for me because of that, kind of, well, my mom stayed at home with my sisters and me, and so I think there was a lot of guilt related to that too. **(Karen)**

Paula also discussed the negative impact of adhering to powerful social constructs regarding motherhood.

I had to be supermom, and I put these incredibly impossible expectations and unrealistic expectations on myself, and I would just beat myself up. It felt like I could not escape this. You felt like everywhere you turned, you saw this, like, gorgeous mom holding a newborn, with her hair perfect instead of having bags under her eyes, and a burp cloth, and wearing, like, yesterday's—you know, maybe she's still in her pajamas or yoga pants, and maybe, maybe she got a shower. It's, like, come on! That's really what it should look like. **(Paula)**

Similarly, Georgia recognized her own new and powerful constructs of motherhood after PPD.

I love my kids, and I actively chose to be a mother. But they're not the be-all-and-the-end-all of my life. They enrich my life, and I love being their mother, and I love watching them grow up. But they're not like my purpose. Of course, that's just a very, very personal thing. But I do think, I think it's important that more and more of us manifest that. Like, "I love my kids, but sometimes I fucking hate being a mother." Like, let's be honest. I am equally as worthy of being factored into the equation. I don't, I don't sacrifice myself on the altar of my children. **(Georgia)**

Postpartum depression made women aware of how they were holding unrealistic beliefs about motherhood. In its devastating impact, PPD gave women no choice but to be "imperfect"—to face the reality of perfect motherhood as anything but reality. Women were thankful they got to let that go, and they were not looking back. The good mother myth died during untreated PPD.

I often say that one of the gifts of motherhood, and certainly of postpartum depression, was that I let go of some of the very strict standards that I held myself to. I no longer feel like I have to compete with—not necessarily that anyone is setting me up for that feeling, but sometimes we can set ourselves up, or expectations of being the most creative, amazing, involved mom and I kind of let things go a little bit . . . I joke sometimes that the title of my autobiography will be, "No, I Don't Iron My Sheets and Other Crimes Against Humanity." **(Anna)**

Do I make my own baby food? Do I do disposable diapers or cloth diapers? All those stupid little choices that don't really make a difference in your relationship with your child were really overwhelming for me. I always thought there was something wrong with me because I didn't enjoy the demands of an infant. I just— I mean, I loved my daughters. I would stare at them for hours. I loved the way they smelled. I loved the way they could fall asleep on my chest. I loved all that. But I hate the baby stage. I hate it! I don't ever want to do it again, and I'm okay with that.

People look at me like I have ten heads when I say it because moms aren't supposed to say stuff like that, I guess. There isn't a discussion around having those. So, you start really thinking that there's something majorly wrong with you if you don't completely lose your identity as an individual and devote everything to your child at all costs. **(Haley)**

The knowledge of having been through PPD informed women that compassion for self, self-care, and honesty were crucial components to sustaining transformation, new beliefs and attitudes about motherhood were created, and old patterns were accepted. Georgia reflected:

> *I still have my Type A temperament. I'll never get rid of that. But perfectionism? Fuck it. Maybe that's just me; maybe that's just motherhood. But I just don't have time or energy for that anymore. And that is such a huge gift because that's no way to live your life. Living a life . . . women were telling me about living.* **(Georgia)**

Living a life that had been threatened by postpartum depression, women realized a commitment to living that life authentically, realistically, and fully grew from living through the worst thing that had ever happened to them. Within the new confidence and honesty, women also reported phenomenal changes in compassion for others.

More Compassionate and Less Judgmental

Remarkably, every woman interviewed talked about an increased compassion or empathy for others that they didn't have before PPD. They frequently used the variations of the word give, given, and giving in describing how PPD had given them compassion.

> *Going through this experience has now allowed me to relate to other people that have gone through it. It has given me compassion and empathy.* **(Mindy)**

> *Oh, I'm definitely less judgmental. Like, before you have kids, you're like, "Oh my God, when I'm a mom, I'll never do that." And then you have kids, and you're like, "Oh my God, anything that it takes, I will do." As I get older and I see things, and I come through the*

things that I've come through life, I think I've become much more open-minded to things, and like I'm like, "Okay, you do that. I don't really agree, but that's fine with me." **(Diana)**

I really feel like I became, like, a much more compassionate person, and way, way less judgmental. Like, a good example of that is there was a mom in the group who formula-fed, and she told us, "You know what, I don't like breastfeeding. I can breastfeed, but I don't want to do it. I don't like it. So, this is what I'm doing." And, you know, I found myself being totally fine with that. Before, I would have really been judge-y toward her, but now I was just, like, "You go, girl. You do whatever you got to do." **(Jamie)**

Not only did women see themselves as less judgmental and more compassionate, but they saw this change in caring for others as a gift. Here, the language of suffering became the language of gratitude for having suffered and a deep understanding of the suffering of others.

I'd like to say if PPD gave me anything, it was definitely an understanding of depression. I look around now at people, and I just have a whole different view: "This person must be suffering from depression." Or I think of people in jail, and how their lives have been destroyed, and how many of them must be suffering from mental disorders or depression, and just couldn't get help for it. **(Vicki)**

I'm a social worker, and it's given me much greater empathy. I have greater empathy about the resources that my clients don't have, and yet they have survived from the same thing. When I feel I am really struggling, I think of my clients and think of what they've gone through and survived. They had it worse, and they still survived and are moving on. **(Janis)**

Everyone talks about my empathy level and what I've been through to cause me to have such an empathic nature. And I do believe that. I think I was an empathic person before, just naturally, but I definitely think that my experiences with PPD have made me more empathetic. **(Faith)**

I'm realizing that I don't really know what it's like to live in anybody else's shoes, or walk down anybody else's path, except mine. I'm a big advocate now of, "do what you need to do." You know? Like, use the tools that you need because we're lucky enough to live in a society where we have access to those tools, including meds and whatever else you need. So, we should be able to use them then and not feel like guilty about it. I think that change was huge. **(Karen)**

Unpacking Stigma

Living through untreated PPD allowed women to recognize and reconcile previously internalized stigma of mental illness. For some, like Callie, the experience revealed a hidden stigma regarding her use of medication.

I really, truly thought when I started to heal from postpartum depression, I could get off of medication because I was on a concoction. I had an antidepressant, lithium, and antipsychotic. I had that right combination that gave me that stability at the time. And then as I became well and whole, I got right off the antidepressant, I got right off the lithium. And then I was going to get off the last one, the antipsychotic, and everything, whoa. I had that internalized stigma where I truly thought like getting off medication means I'm cured. I'm well. And I didn't realize that stigma. And I don't relate to it now because the last medication, the antipsychotic, I need that. I have no problem taking that. And I thank God that we have medications. I explain it to people,

I mean, you have a cold, you take Tylenol. You have cancer, and you might have chemo or surgery. Thank God that we're in a world where we have access to these things and that it's continuing to be fine-tuned. And yes, is it a perfect world? No. But I'm of the mindset that it's about how you relate to things and how you know yourself that help you make those choices for yourself. And I can't tell you what's right for you. But I'm grateful that we have these options available to us. **(Callie)**

It's made me a lot more compassionate to what other people are going through, especially mental illness. I have a whole new understanding of all kinds of mental passive-aggressive, but especially depression.

I'm more compassionate towards anybody's plight, towards any illness, cancer. I have more compassion in me for other people, and I want to help other people in any way that I can, but especially moms, because that's exactly what I went through. I have a greater understanding of mental illness, and like my grandmother, who was schizophrenic, you know, I never really quite understood either, and now I just, you know, it breaks my heart that she never really got to live a normal life. **(Sienna)**

It was certainly never an experience that I would wish on anybody, and I was very relieved not to have it the second time around, but I will say that it totally did change me as a person and make me appreciate, you know I think the whole field of mental health a lot more. I mean, my viewpoints on mental health changed, I'll tell you that.

You know, it's so embarrassing, but, like, I remember—I had had a couple of miscarriages, and it really made me feel like I needed to treat pregnancy like it was this holy miraculous thing. But, you know, then I was there, right there, being exactly in the place that I thought I would never be—suffering with a mental illness. And you know, that's really humbling. **(Betsy)**

Betsy's description of the humbling shift in a compassionate attitude toward others who have mental illness was followed by her discussion of the increased confidence developed through PPD. Women's experience after PPD included powerful indicators of change. (See Figure 4.)

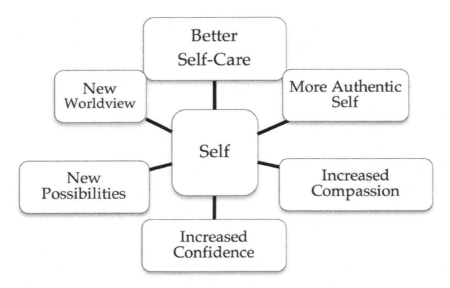

Fig 4: Representation of the Components of Transformed Sense of Self

The transition of seeing self-transformed in the world evolved into a perception of others as safe. Assumptions of the world as benevolent were formed, and women felt safe to engage in the world. Anna's words summarize.

PPD does help you kind of break down your assumptions about people, and it is a great leveler. Women I never would have thought of becoming close friends within my life before postpartum. And now they're a very interwoven part of my life. **(Anna)**

PART 2: TRANSFORMED RELATIONSHIPS

A stabilized assumption of the world as benevolent was correlated with women building new beliefs about their world as again making sense. For many, this paradigm shift resulted from women transforming relationships that were no longer serving them after PPD. To create an assumptive world that made sense, women reassessed relationships with partners, the family of origin, and friends.

Partners

Relationships were a significant part of the way women saw themselves transformed after PPD. Not surprisingly, women described significant changes in their relationships with their partners.

> *PPD made our relationship stronger, the fact that he would support me and be with me through everything. I don't take that for granted at all.* **(Haley)**

> *While there were some very difficult times, it really only served to strengthen our marriage and our partnership. I don't know if that would have happened if we hadn't gone through that. I think it ultimately brought us closer together.* **(Anna)**

> *Through it all, he supported, and he witnessed me in my pain and in my struggle, and you know he was always there. He never doubted me for a minute. I would tell him, "I'm not supposed to be a mom. This was a big mistake. This was a big mistake." And he was always so confident in me, and he would always say, "No, no, you're good. You'll get it." And he was right. And I think, if open-minded, it deepened our relationship, you know, just going through such a hard time together. It was like being in a war together or being in*

a foxhole together. You're really bonded on a deeper level. He and I are much kinder to each other. We're much gentler with each other. We didn't fight very much before, but we haven't had a fight since my son was born. So, I think we're just very, like, careful and gentle with each other, having been through PPD. **(Jamie)**

Having struggled with fertility due to PCOS, Deborah's journey with her husband took on new significance in light of her PPD.

I spent all of this effort and all of this emotion, and you know, I thought this was what I wanted, I thought this was what I wanted, I thought this, and then my baby is defective, and I don't like this, and oh my god, I did this to us, and it's going to destroy my marriage. You know, all of those things. I mean, so many people get divorced in that process of infertility and all of that, and somehow my husband managed to take it in stride as much as he could. He had been with me through bouts of depression before, so it wasn't that he was totally unused to me being altered at different points depending on stressors, but this was huge. I mean, my transition from zero to one was really, really hard. And then the added layer of I feel so guilty because I worked so hard to have this happen. **(Deborah)**

For others, the transformation of relationships with partners after PPD was divorce.

We went to therapy for about a year and a half, until I said, "No, I'm done." I could see myself changing during that process, and then completely changing after we separated. In terms of it being transformative, when I think of that, I think, like, absolutely it was! **(Beatrice)**

I'm moving forward. I continue to take steps forward in my life. I've separated from my husband, and I don't look at that as a bad thing because right now, I'm working on finding who I am, and recognizing that I can't be in any kind of relationship unless I'm happy with me. **(Mindy)**

I look back at it because everything has changed. I'm divorced now. And he has custody of the children. I'm still involved as much as I can be. We Skype every week. Ultimately, what led to our divorce was that he had addiction issues, and now I look back on my postpartum experiences, and I can't help but wonder if it was really me, or if it was the fact that he was struggling with addiction and then that weighed on our marriage. **(Sandy)**

My husband is an alcoholic, and he had stopped drinking. And then all this happened. Shortly after my PPD, I found out that he had an affair during that time. The affair was like a step back. And then, once I had found out about the affair, and I divorced him, and then he started drinking again. You know, my husband went through this with me, but he ended up not able to cope, and we got the divorce.

We were divorced for five years. But then, two years ago, we got back together. So, we're still continuing this healing journey. The relationship he had to me was feeling like I left like I was completely gone. And he felt helpless to help me and didn't know that I was ever coming back. I can say, though, that process, I know my strengths, and I didn't before. I know my worth and a lot of things had to change in my relationship with my ex-husband.

Right now, we're building a home, and we have six acres. My five-year plan is I'm building an octagonal space that people can come and use for meditation, Tai Chi, yoga in our home with me and my now ex-husband, boyfriend, soon to be husband again, and two children. It's symbolic of our journey together and what we're building and the stability of what we're building now. And it's a really beautiful process. (Callie)

Family of Origin

Changes in relationships with members of women's families of origin were also characterized as transformed by several women.

My relationship with my mom improved after PPD, which is sort of an upside to it. And that didn't happen until much later, when she read my book, and she called me in tears, and she was like, "Oh my God, I had no idea that you were going through that. I feel like I failed you because I didn't recognize it." And I didn't feel that way at all. **(Betsy)**

I really started taking the very scary step of interacting differently with my family, my family of origin, so my parents and my sister. Really being able to say, use my feeling words. **(Paula)**

For Janis, her unique experience as an identical twin became central component of her experience of transformed relationships after PPD. In describing her relationship with her twin sister, Janis shared:

We're very similar. We both do the same field of work, and we went to college together. We have a lot of similarities at home. In many ways, it's more intimate than my relationship with my husband and my relationship with my parents. I don't have any other siblings, so I don't know how the relationship is with a non-twin. But I experienced postpartum depression, and she didn't. That was difficult because even though really going through my hardest time, she couldn't understand. So that has been a big transformation in my relationships. Over the years, something about my postpartum depression just changed the relationship, and it allowed me an appreciation of each other in a better, different way. **(Janis)**

Friendships

Many women also reported changes in friendships. Betsy experienced an evolution in her relationship with her mother, while simultaneously experiencing the ending of a relationship with a lifelong best friend.

> *I don't think I even tried to talk to her about it because I felt like there was no way in hell she would understand. I just couldn't. I don't think I could go there with her, and I think that was the first step down. Our closeness really dissipated after that. At this point, I consider her a casual friend, and that is crazy, considering I talked to her more than I talked to my parents. Here was my best friend, who was supposed to know me better than anyone, and even she didn't want to hear it.* **(Betsy)**

While Betsy experienced the loss of a meaningful friendship held before PPD, other women reported gaining new friendships after PPD.

> *I have forged new relationships, new friendships that I didn't have before.* **(Haley)**

> *Women I never would have thought of becoming close friends within my life before postpartum. And now they're a very interwoven part of my life.* **(Anna)**

PART 3: TRANSFORMED SELF IN THE WORLD

One of the most significant ways women saw themselves changed by PPD was in considering new possibilities for themselves in the world. They felt worthy of being a part of their transformed world in new and meaningful ways. Women considered new possibilities for themselves in the world: (a) new career, (b) returning to school, (c) professional or vocational change, (d) writing or creativity, and (d) advocacy. For example, seven of the 25 women returned to school, four women published their first book, five women started blogs, two started non-profits, and two began entirely new careers. The sense of self as worthy took on a positive mindset of potential and purpose, just as Grace shares.

> *One of the big changing moments in my life after this experience was realizing that I had very much a fixed mindset before. And now, I have a growth mindset. And I thought I only had certain abilities, and I thought I like to do certain things and had a certain intelligence.*
>
> *Now I see that's completely not true, and I value the strengths that I do have that I always downplayed in the past before this happened, so much more. So, things like being sensitive, being observant, connecting deeply, understanding things on a different level that most people wouldn't. I always thought those were "soft skills." But I realized how important they are. You know, the further in life I get, I realize how important those are.* **(Grace)**

Career

Remarkably, 100% of the women reported changing career or professional paths in some manner and attributed the change to their experience of PPD. For example, Beatrice said:

> *It changed my entire professional path. I decided to go back to psychotherapy as a postpartum depression specialist. I had left the field*

for ten years, and part of the reason why is because I went through postpartum depression. It definitely was the impetus to think, "I can do this. I think I can go back and be a therapist again." **(Beatrice)**

Part of my transformation was totally changing my career. I left behind a career in journalism that I loved. I am actually in the course of becoming a clinical social worker and doing the work that I do now as a therapist and that I've done in the recent past as a researcher. I think in some ways, transformation is going to be happening for the rest of my life. Oh my God, I am really so thankful for it every day. **(Georgia)**

An ad came on TV for this school saying, "We have a new dental hygiene program." And I was like, "All right, well, I'll call!" I was scared to death, to death, but I was like, "I can do this, I have to do this. Like, I have to." I mean, I went back to school! I remember when I was scared to leave the living room, and here I am. I'm back at school. I have a 4.0. I'm class president. School has been the best experience for me. It's been amazing. **(Diana)**

I became a postpartum doula two and a half years ago. So, I worked as a certified nursing assistant at our local hospital for nine years in various settings. And then I was a stay-at-home mom for a while. And knowing that I wanted to do that, but also feeling like I needed some other type of purpose and not really knowing. Like, and I really knowing. Like, and I really enjoy taking care of people. Like, I thought I was going to be a nurse at one point, and then realizing that that was not how I wanted to take care of people. When I found being a postpartum doula, which I didn't even know was a thing until very shortly before I became one. Just knowing that's what I wanted to do, to be able to take care of somebody. **(Grace)**

Helena also started a career as a postpartum doula, and eventually returned to school for licensure as a mental health counselor specializing in working with women who have experienced PPD.

It was a very conscious effort of—it was part of my treatment plan that I was making for myself to help other people to become a doula, to become a mover and a shaker in the birth community. That was a very conscious part of my healing. It still is. It still drives who I am. I still literally feel, sitting in the chair of the therapist now, like moms who are struggling, how important it is to just bear witness to their struggles, to let them know "you're not alone," to let them know, "I'm not walking your shoes, but I've walked that path with you, and you're not alone." **(Helena)**

Jamie, a tech industry professional, returned to graduate school to become a licensed mental health professional.

I worked in the tech industry. I tested software for a living. I always had a desire to change my career path to work in mental health in some capacity. Before my son was born, I wondered why I hadn't gone back to school yet. Since my experience with PPD, I know I am in the right place at the right time. Had I entered the mental health profession before I went through all of this, I would not have nearly as much to give to people. **(Jamie)**

Skye expressed a sense of transformation in becoming a mental health counselor.

I think the big difference this time, at this point in my life, is that I am a counselor now, who works with pregnant and postpartum moms. I've really been able to heal myself a lot through the work I do with other moms. Seeing myself in them and realizing that, you know, it wasn't me. I do feel like the things that I've come through, they really changed me. They changed me on every level. **(Skye)**

Janis explained that through the experience of PPD, she realized that she needed to change her position at work.

*I've changed jobs. I left the position that I had been in for three
years before my daughter was born. It's the position I got right
out of grad school, and it was the job I returned to after my maternity leave. I realized that it was not pleasing for me any longer.
It was not the work I wanted to be doing. I had to make a change
and leave the position to make more changes in the way I was
interacting with my work, and I've been able to do that.* **(Janis)**

Writing

Thirteen of the 25 women expressed that some form of writing
about PPD was an extension of their transformation in the world.

*After I wrote my book, I did a few activities around that. It was kind
of like that's how I made peace with it, and I moved on.* **(Dana)**

*I put everything—all my experiences, all my thoughts, everything—
into what became hundreds of pages. It took me a very long
time to put it in an order that made sense. I always look back at
my own writing and think, "Wow, I can't believe I wrote that."
The process of educating myself through books and articles, getting
all my thoughts and feelings out onto paper, putting it together
in a way that made sense, working with a creative team to publish it,
re-reading it at times, and sharing it with other people, helped
to transform me.* **(Morgan)**

*I just really wanted to refocus myself. But then, once he was born
and PPD happened, I started journaling. Once I got better, I got
really angry about a lot of things about how we're treated as women
postpartum and prenatally. And that kind of provoked me to switch
gears, become a blogger, write a book, and start trying to reach out*

to other women who had had PPD to make sure they didn't feel as, like, alone and lost, and scared as I had. **(Betsy)**

I think that PPD helped transform how I think about what I do—that's a big piece of my transformation. I work for the state. And when I first came back to work, I started looking at what are we doing at the state level related to postpartum depression or anything related to that. I wrote a grant along with another woman. The grant is to implement mother-infant therapy groups into home visiting programs around the state. It was pretty awesome. That's another way that I helped myself get through some of that—being able to channel it into something that I knew how to do and could work towards. **(Vicki)**

Even in the psych hospital, all I wanted was to talk to another mom because I was the only mom there! After I got better, I looked into seeing if there were any resources for moms in my area, and there weren't. So, I started a webpage and started a support group. I think working with other moms, in the beginning, gave me something to focus on. It gave me energy outside of myself. I realized I can help these people. I can educate myself. I can help women find the resources that they need, so they don't have to fall as far as I did.

I can't tell you how many times, especially [online] that I've heard, "I am so happy that you're doing this. I'm so happy that this community exists because I know that I can get on any time of day or night and not be alone." For me, that's huge. There's this community that exists all because I went through hell. And for me, that makes it worth it. **(Sandy)**

I really, honestly, a lot of it was inspired by some of the moms that I met online, women like Ivy Shih Leung, and after reading her book, it was kind of like, "Wow, I feel empowered, and I want to be able to share my story when it's appropriate, and tell people my struggles."

I've always loved writing, and I had forgotten how much I enjoyed it and how much I enjoyed being creative. So, it took me a while to figure out how to get everything set up; then I took the plunge, probably about the spring of this past year. I've been able to help people who are struggling kind of see themselves in what I'm writing. **(Paula)**

Advocacy

So, after the first year, I decided that I was going to start volunteering and giving back and really feeling like it was so important for people to understand that they don't have to go through it, or if they are going through it, that there are people that can help. That's when I really started to feel the power from it and the transformation.

When I started facilitating support groups and, like, every time somebody would talk, it gave a little more meaning to what I went through. Just chipping away at the negativity behind it all, which was really awesome. You know, I went through this, but it doesn't have to be fully negative and that I can make it into something to help other people and to help myself feel better. **(Grace)**

I started a nonprofit to hopefully change the educational landscape around perinatal mental health. I have so many ideas. I really don't know. I want to continue sharing my story. I feel like I'm transitioning into the education side and not so much the sharing. It's been a phenomenal year. It really has. **(Margery)**

Part of my healing journey, initially, in earlier years, I volunteered, and I helped support other women. I wrote an article about my experience. I started forming local support groups and building communities locally.

Then, part of the healing was realizing that I no longer identify with this, and I have to let that go too. And so, I did. I'm still in touch with different people that I met through that process, where I was blessed to help when I was coming full circle. Me helping them was part of my healing. **(Callie)**

Conclusion

The understanding of self-care as a mechanism of deserving to exist was experienced through increased compassion for self and others. Understanding the suffering of PPD extended women's ability to contextualize themselves in their world, and in the world relative to others. Surviving the suffering of the during dimension of untreated PPD enabled a self-confidence not previously known. Old schemas of self, destroyed through the experience of PPD, gave way to new schemas of possibilities in relationships, professional, and vocational aspirations. The women were different people and continue to experience change as a result of their suffering.

I'm still transforming in smaller ways, you know, the healing, we talk about healing, as a lot of people talk about is the spiral, right? It's not a straight line, because it's never, you know, from here to there, and you're done, and it's not messy. Healing is very messy.

And you kind of come around the same thing over and over and say, "Wow, didn't I learn my lesson about that, you know, that taking care of myself, or setting boundaries, or, you know, advocating for what I need in the moment?" And then you finally realize, "Yes, but I'm doing it in a different level now. Like it's a deeper level or at a higher level of understanding that I'm still transforming." It may be smaller in terms of the magnitude of that transformation. But for me, I still think it's going. **(Adrienne)**

The momentum for this growth was generated by self-confidence and strength gained from struggling to survive through PPD.

And the momentum continued the process of transformation beyond recovery or resilience. As we see in the next chapter, there was something else going on here: women reported a dimension of transformation that included existential purpose.

CHAPTER 6

BEYOND POSTPARTUM DEPRESSION: PARADOX AND PURPOSE

Someone I loved once gave me a box full of darkness.
It took me years to understand that
this too, was a gift.

– Mary Oliver –

T he data gathered described being unprepared before PPD, shattered during PPD, and the specific ways women were changed after PPD. But there was more. Women went on, sharing experiences of change beyond recovery and resilience. Women described surviving untreated PPD as a paradox that birthed a purpose greater than themselves, transforming perspectives on life itself. The transformation extended women existentially, infusing them with a sense of wanting to put their wisdom to work in the world.

PARADOX: WHY DID IT HAPPEN?

Every woman I interviewed reported that living through un-treated PPD was the hardest, worst, or most difficult thing they'd ever experienced—and that they had each been transformed by it in significant, positive, and meaningful ways. For many, this began with an intrapersonal questioning as to why they experienced suffering, and what the meaning of their struggling to survive was.

For me, it was almost like just breaking. PPD broke all the all the bad stuff open, but it broke all the good stuff open as well. And once everything was sort of on the table, I felt like it was an opportunity to rearrange all the pieces and put them back in a way that makes sense for me now, which is different, looks a lot different, I feel, than what it was before this experience, and how I look at them. **(Grace)**

Part of my transformation was at first, like okay, I went through this. It was really hard, and what can I appreciate out of it? My goal is to try and find appreciation in things that happen to me. So instead of letting them be—dwelling on them or being this horrible side, what can I pull from this and give it appreciation? **(Mindy)**

I think, about on a very spiritual level, I wondered what was happening? Was I going through some kind of rebirth, and that's why it was so traumatic? **(Haley)**

I'm 42 years old, how do I parse out what's a result of this experience, and the transformation that I went through, and continue to go through? For me, a healthy portion of it is the healing, the transformation that I experienced directly as a result of my PPD, and of the help that I was able to seek. Now, I don't need it anymore. I am who I am. I'm somebody who has suffered from mental illness, and I will call it that. **(Georgia)**

Georgia's new understanding of the transformation directly resulting from her experience of PPD was echoed by many.

I felt like, "Okay, why did I feel like I wasn't a good mom when my child was one, but by the time he was four, I felt like I was a really good mom? I'm still the same person, so what is the difference there?" It has to be that this depression really changed the way I viewed myself and viewed the situation. **(Haley)**

I believe I was meant to experience postpartum depression. I don't know why; I just know that I came out a different person. I'm a survivor and proud of it. I keep telling myself if I could survive postpartum depression, I could survive most anything. Sure, I lost precious bonding time with my daughter during the weeks I was sick with PPD. But I decided to make the most of my PPD experience. I have accepted what's happened to me—I have no regrets. **(Morgan)**

I guess the word that comes to mind for me is "astonishing." And that, I think that word encompasses a lot of what I feel about it. For me, that something or so many good things could come from probably, one of the worst experiences of my life. When you think about it, if I had gone up to the top of to that building? I wouldn't be here. I would be dead (I subsequently found out).

I think, wow, everyone that I'm close to, all of my siblings and subsequently, the people that they're close to, I mean, everyone is transformed. Everyone's transformed by it because they saw it, and they know (a) that it happens, and (b) that you don't need to just, like, sit by and watch it happen, and not do anything about it. **(Georgia)**

It's a bittersweet blessing. But I feel like it's a blessing that I'm supposed to use. It makes me feel good about myself because it makes me feel like I'm giving back. I just feel like I'm paying it forward, I guess you would say. **(Faith)**

I know you hear a lot of women say that "I wouldn't wish it on my worst enemy" (and I wouldn't wish it my worst enemy), but I have learned to look back at the experience as a gift, as a time of tremendous growth because I honestly think that I needed it to become the person that I am today. It really did trigger a tremendous amount of growth in my life. So, the way I see it, I've been given this gift. Yeah, it kind of sucks to be depressed and need to go to the psychiatric hospital, but on the other hand, it's taught me a lot about life, living, and how to take care of myself, and how to—it's given me the ability to help others to take care of them as well. **(Sandy)**

PURPOSE: PUTTING WISDOM TO WORK IN THE WORLD

Wondering how and why they experienced the trauma of untreated PPD revealed an abiding change in women's worldviews. Women put their wisdom to work for the benefit of others in powerful ways: writing books, blogs, grants, hosting online support groups, Twitter chats, creating photography and videography projects to increase awareness, volunteering to facilitate support groups, reaching out to coworkers suffering with PPD, joining PPD organizations, helping other mothers, and volunteering to participate in this study. As Sandy, now a highly successful PPD advocate with a large community, explained:

But there's this community that exists, all because I went through hell. And for me, that makes it worth it. If one mom needs help and I help at least one mom, then I've achieved my goal for the day. And that's a good thing. **(Sandy)**

Using the experience as a tool to help others were ways women experienced their transformation currently. Vicki shared:

I know it kind of sounds bad, but I use it. I use my experience to relate to people. So, for example, some of my work in public health, I really care a lot about the issues in the world, like racism, and sexism, and classism. And I think equality for people is so important. And I hope to, you know, not using it in a negative way, but use it in a way that this needs to stop. This lack of support for each other, from mental illness to if people can't afford something that they need, like, clothes, or food, or homes, like those things, this lack of being able to do that. That is what I want to—and I don't know a better to say that but use that for. **(Vicki)**

Mindy described an experience in a mother's support group, during which she realized the need to use her experience for the benefit of others.

I would sit in this room, and I'm like, "Is no one experiencing the same thing I am? I'm struggling here" . . . everyone's, like, "Oh, but don't struggle. You might struggle, but you got to appreciate these moments because you won't have these moments for very long. Your kids will get old, and then you'll regret it." And I'm, like, "I just want someone who can just say, 'Yes, this is fucking hard.'" So, through this, I decided I am going to be that person. I feel that's why we have to go through these things. **(Mindy)**

I don't think you can have an experience that is that massive in terms of resulting in a personal paradigm shift. I don't think you can have something like that recede into the background. I think every woman who has a chance to speak about the experience can help others.

And for me, especially to be able to tag onto that experience, the positivity that came out of it at the end is a message that I'm happy to share and circulate again and again. I think it's really important for women and their families, really, who have experienced this, or yet to experience it, to also know that as dark as it can be, that for many of us, there's a very, very light side of it that can come afterward.

It's a lost opportunity if you don't do that, if you don't use that kind of situation to help others. I mean, at least to help yourself, to be able to see it for what it is, and really spend some time thinking about it, and how has it changed me as a person; that's great, and that's important, that I almost feel like it's an obligation.

We're never given a situation that we truly can't handle, even if at the moment, it feels that way. And that once you scale your biggest barrier, everything else in comparison is easier. And that's generally been my attitude over these last six years. Like, as miserable as it is for each of us to go through this, if we don't do anything to write about it, or talk about it, or reach out to other women, we're just kind of failing on a fundamental requirement of womanhood, almost. But for those people who have been blessed enough to have made some sort of transition, or had the ability to gain some insight, then to me that's the next obvious step, to turn it around and try to do, make some good out of it. **(Dana)**

Helena, now a licensed psychotherapist working with women who suffer from perinatal and postpartum mood and anxiety disorders, described how she uses her own experience of PPD as a guide from which she guides others to healing.

This past year, I've been, at times, just trying to sit in the fire when it comes. Sit with the darkness and the scariness, and say, and try to say, "Okay, what is this informing me? Does it mean my life is up in arms, and it's a really big sign that I need to do a course correction," as opposed to just avoiding that feeling? Encouraging my clients in the same way toward trying to turn towards it as a sign, as a beacon for, "Okay, you're out of whack in something, and your life has a— there's something that's a mineral deficiency, so to speak, and let's figure out whether it is so that we can improve your health again."

I think I will be transforming for a lifetime because it is one of those formative events that makes like a tree growing out of a boulder. You know you have to—the roots are still in the cracks, and yet, they're stabilizing you at the same time. And you're growing, you might, your trunk might bend, but you grow into a mentor, and then you grow up straight. I do feel like I'm growing towards the light. I've corrected the balance, per se, even though you're always making adjustments. But my roots are in those cracks. That's what forms my entire orientation to what I do. **(Helena)**

For Sienna, her awareness to use her experience to help others evolved from an experience at church.

The first time I went back to church, I was probably six weeks postpartum and still in the depths of it, and I had heard his message, and his message was listen, if you have struggled with something or are struggling with something, don't let your struggles be in vain. It is, like, you need to reach out and help people. And there's nobody that can help other people unless they've gone through the exact same situation.

And his example was rape, like, there's nobody that can help somebody that's been raped as well as another person who's been raped. Or somebody who's experienced a psychiatric illness, you know, especially like—I took it as God was speaking through him as a message to me that I need to use this experience, this devastating experience, to help other people, other moms that may be suffering. **(Sienna)**

Mindy described an awareness of her transformation through putting her experience to work in a photography project.

It wasn't until I did that project where I was able to I think fully positively transform in my life, and move forward, because I realized, at that point, I didn't have to be stuck in these feelings, that that was part of my life, part of my pregnancy, part of my childbirth experience, but it didn't have to define me as a person . . . [Inaudible] when I could laugh about it and share it and cry about it. It allowed me to move.

Also, it made me aware that this was such an important topic for all women. What I went through, what these women went through, none of us want anyone else to experience this alone. If we can stop people from experiencing it, I think, hands down, all of us would do anything we could to stop any woman from having this experience. **(Mindy)**

Georgia left a successful career as a journalist to become a licensed clinical social worker following her experience with PPD. She also now volunteers as a support group leader and advocate. She noted that she was aware of her continuing to transform in this way.

Every mom that I meet transforms me a little bit more as I learn about their experiences, and how similar, but different, what we call "PPD" or postpartum depression, how different it can be. Interacting with these moms reinforce, for me, my own transformation. It, like, manifests, it, like, reflects it back to me. And so, therefore, makes it all the more real, and the more solid, solidifying it or, I don't know, I'm having this visualization of myself being, like, I was saying kind of always in transformation, so maybe, not totally, like, whole. And each mom that I meet, like, adds another piece to me that is this post-postpartum person. **(Georgia)**

Faith explained that she is aware of the ways her transformation has extended into her current life, 13 years after PPD in similar ways.

I think through sharing with other people, I do. Because if I speak or write about my experiences, it's like I gain new insight as to how I was able to transform the way I have or how I continue to transform from the experiences. **(Faith)**

Sandy described:

You know you hear about people who have died and seen the light and gone toward it and, like, given up? Then they come back, and

174

they have a second chance. So, this coming back from falling so far from what's expected to be normal and falling so far from good mental health, it just makes you grateful for every day that you have. Even when the days are hard, you know, it isn't as hard as the days back then. It's not as dark. (Sandy)

Callie noted:

It's like wisdom. Until you embody something, and then you allow it, and you have the strength to allow it to wash through you, you don't know it. And so that's what I was able to do.

The image that came to me was kind of me having this personality that was kind of almost like a web around my spirit. My spirit and my truth and who I really was always broke through that. It was trying to break free, but there was still like a web of me holding myself like kind of protecting myself.

And I love who I am. I can laugh at my personality traits that I contend with. But the difference is, back then, I was serving myself, and I was serving my ego. Now, my spirit is serving me. **(Callie)**

Perception: Sensation and Intuition

Many women described experiencing meaningful coincidences and events regarding their connection to others. The nature of this component of the dimension of beyond PPD was one of new or unique extrasensory perception not previously experienced. Women did not report finding these occurrences alarming, distressing, or remarkable, but a part of their awareness of ways they had experienced transformation.

Mindy, for example, shared her encounter with a coincidence regarding the work on her photo project about PPD. She had enrolled in a photography class following her PPD and went to discuss topics for a final project with her professor. She shared:

*And then, it was funny, and that might be why that photo project
came up at the same time because I believe that things aren't really coincidental, things come into our life for a reason. I said when
I tapped on that classroom, and I'm, like, postpartum depression.
I'm, like, "Where in the hell did that come from? Why did that
topic come to mind?" But it did, right at that moment.* **(Mindy)**

Mindy's experience of sudden suggestion created a new perception
of both the import of her transformation and the possibility of
purposing wisdom gained through suffering through her creativity. The experience of developed wisdom through increased
perception for many came through their relationships with their
babies. Although more subtle, women spoke of the paradox of
having extraordinary bonds with children and also having struggled so greatly with PPD during the early stages of motherhood.
Betsy explained her sense of the connection with her son.

*But there's—I don't know, this feeling of, "We were in this battle
together, and we both have these war wounds, and we share that
common bond." Whereas, like, when I had Lucy, it was, you know,
just pure joy, and fun, and wonderful, and that's great too. It's just
different.* **(Betsy)**

Realization of differences in one's ability to bond and the quality of
the bond was a perception woman developed through the suffering of PPD. For Jamie, this came in the form of a different kind
of bond with her son than she had anticipated prior to PPD.

*I think for me, the key part of it is this idea of intentionality. I thought
that when I had a baby that I would, you know, I would love him
right away and that everything would just come naturally, including birthing, and it didn't.*

*And, you know, I think one thing that was part of this whole trans-
formative feeling that my postpartum depression gave me was that
I've come to believe that there are times in our life where we love*

*somebody because we just do, and we just fall in love with them, or
we fall in love with the situation or something like that. And there
are times when we really have to be intentional and say I am going
to work really hard to make love grow here.*

*And I've found that doing that produces a love that is no less genu-
ine than the kind that just comes, sort of generates on its own. And
that it feels stronger to me because my bond with my son feels very
strong to me because I had to work to get it.* **(Jamie)**

Jamie confronted the loss of assumptions held before motherhood. Jamie realized that loving a child took work, and intention
to "make love grow here." The wisdom gained beyond that realization was that the value of love that is worked on, nurtured, and
intentionally purposed, was no less than the preconceived ideal
of love held before PPD. Moreover, the strength of the bond with
her son resulted because of the work she put into creating it. In
this way, the experience of struggling through PPD generated a
bond with her son stronger than what she had imagined before
PPD, encountered during, or experienced in the after dimensions
of transformation through PPD.

Dana also described a sense of connection with her son
beyond what she had with her other children, due to their experiencing the struggle to survive PPD together.

*But the other thing that was interesting is I felt at the time my
son's birth, and to continue to feel that I have a different bond
with him than with my other kids, which, of course, I could never
admit to them. But because he and I went through that together
and survived the pregnancy, despite my wishes otherwise in the
beginning. A lot of people will think it's just a thing inside of you
that has nothing to do with it. But I really came to feel like that's
where the partnership was. That it wasn't just me deciding to*

change my mind, and it wasn't just him having to survive. But it was something we survived together. **(Dana)**

The partnership of survival Dana described was a dimension of the transformation through PPD that extended the experience beyond recovery, or the ending of her symptoms. She was aware of the changed quality of the connection to her son.

Other observations of extended or enhanced perceptual capacities were described as awareness of the impact of sharing one's story with a group of people. Georgia described such an experience during a training course following her PPD.

> *There was a day, and it was probably three or so weeks into that eight-week course where I totally broke down, and in the room with these nine strangers and our group leader. But I couldn't keep it together. We were going around the room, talking about bonding with my children, and I just totally fell apart. And it was a scary moment for me because I just remember thinking, like, they're going to reject me.*

> *But there was more interaction among the women. And from that point on, I felt like there was—and when I talked about it since with them because I have gotten to know a lot of them really well, and they kind of felt the same thing, like something changed that day. By sharing what I did, I allowed the other people in the room to just, to be more real about the experience that they were having.* **(Georgia)**

Georgia's perception of the change in the interaction between individuals signified a shift in her perceptual capacities surfacing from, and beyond, her experience of PPD. The sense of increased empathic perception and skill was echoed by Skye, now a counselor working with women who have experienced perinatal mood and anxiety disorders.

> *So, I do feel like the things that I've come through, they really changed me. They changed me on every level to where I can work*

with other women, and I can sense a lot of times what they're going through and how they're feeling. **(Skye)**

Karen also described a sense of transformation among those, with whom she tells her story.

I will talk about it with anybody because, maybe, somewhere along the line, somebody will share it with somebody else, and it'll get to somebody else, and eventually, there will be some better laws, or I don't know, or better support, or another way to look at life. I don't know exactly what it is. But I feel like that is a huge piece of what I want to help support. **(Karen)**

Karen's willingness to share her story as an extension of her growth was echoed by stories and narratives of other women. The ways women described experiencing transformation in their current life included examples of transformed narratives and stories symbolic of the journey.

Anna's story of the pearl earrings described in a previous chapter is another example of this symbolic narrative. When Anna stopped wearing those earrings every day, her friends and family saw it as a visible expression of her transformation. The story, the telling of it, and retelling of it was an extension of her experience beyond recovery. Her narrative of no longer wearing the earring, and not feeling badly about it, signified a profound change in her life story. The story of the pearl earrings became a part of the story of her transformation.

The concept of story was mentioned by Georgia as well. For Georgia, the experience of her story beyond PPD created an awareness of the need for narratives in all aspects of human interaction. Georgia reflected:

You know how in pretty much every culture you know, we have, we have fables, and we have stories that we pass down, and that cultures, that parents tell children and grandparents tell grand-kids. And there's a reason why human beings need to do that. Like, it tells us something about ourselves, and I think that that's what I . . . I think that's what I experience. Like having conversations like this, speaking out to whoever asks me about my experience or individually with the work that I do with the women that I help is to kind of, is to, like, keep this story alive, as painful as it was.

The story is all that I have now of the experience that I had, like the memories, and however, the memories have kind of come together into a story; that's all I have. And so, I think that's why I need to keep myself kind of immersed in it, to remind myself, this is why you are where you are, and doing what you're doing. **(Georgia)**

Sharing stories of symbolic narratives was a component of the description of transforming beyond PPD. For several women, these stories were shared at the end of our interview or after the interview had ended. Diana emailed the following message.

Thank you for listening to my story! It was quite a struggle, but I won! Oh, I was going to mention that the song "Viva La Vida" by Coldplay came out during my suffering, and I related to the lyrics of that so much.

One minute, I held the key

Next, the walls were closed on me

And I discovered that my castles stand

Upon pillars of salt and pillars of sand

It was the wicked and wild wind

Blew down the doors to let me in

Shattered windows and the sound of drums

People couldn't believe what I'd become. **(Diana)**

For Diana, the lyrics made meaning of her experience beyond her own narrative. The words symbolized reflected her suffering, its meaning, and extended her perception of the experience personal description through poetic verse.

Similarly, at the end of our interview, Jamie shared a tremendously significant experience for her regarding her awareness, perception, and sense of transformation by sharing this story. A year after Jamie's PPD, she went to a psychic medium. On her way out of her session, the woman told her to check her phone. Jamie walked to her car, and as instructed, looked at her phone. She recognized the Rumi affirmation feed. The quote for the day was as follows:

I have come,

To drag you out of yourself

And take you into my heart.

I have come

To bring out the beauty

You never knew you had

And lift you like a prayer,

To the sky.

Jamie told me, "I knew in that moment, that was the lesson."

CONCLUSION

I have had many women ask me if I felt transformed as a result of my experience. In reflecting on the lessons of my own experience with PPD, I realized that I did not experience the beyond phase of this process. I think it is important to remember that some women don't find an identifiable existential purpose from the experience. For some, it is an intimacy with death awareness that changes the trajectory of ourselves in the world. Living for the benefit of a child is enough. Staying alive in order to give our children the best shot at life is enough. It is everything.

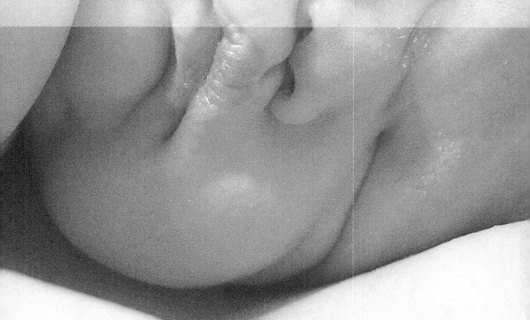

PART II

TRAUMA, TRANSFORMATION, AND POSTPARTUM DEPRESSION: THEORETICAL AND PROFESSIONAL PERSPECTIVE

CHAPTER 7
TRAUMA AND TRANSFORMATION

The wreckage of stars - I built a world
from this wreckage.
– Friedrich Nietzsche –

PPD has been described by women as a journey of suffering and change—wreckage and building. This chapter reflects on how a theory of PPD as traumatic and transformational fits or doesn't fit within established schools of thought on depression. Theoretical comparison triangulates the idea that untreated PPD can be both traumatic and transformative.

Current research acknowledges that PPD co-occurs with confounding factors. The wealth of literature examining risk factors has demonstrated clearly that PPD does not occur in isolation, but rather, in "conjunction with a complex interplay of socio-demographic, biophysical, psychosocial, and behavioral factors" (Jesse & Swanson, 2007, p. 378). Previous history of mental health problems, maternal age, obstetric problems, unplanned pregnancy, lack of social support, violence in the home, and poverty have all been found to increase the risk of PPD.

Health psychologist and trauma expert Kathleen Kendall-Tackett noted that we must consider the social and environmental contexts that women come from, including their families, communities, and cultures. Kendall-Tackett explained,

Women do not become mothers in a vacuum. They live in families, extended families, cultures, and societies. At each of these levels of social connection, mothers can be protected from or made more vulnerable to depression (2010, p. 104).

From this developmental perspective, women are viewed as changing from one state to another through interrelated exposure to and experience with our environment. PPD *develops* relative to multiple intersecting factors. Other theoretical models of depression can expand our thinking about PPD. For example, theories of positive aspects of depression, such as depressive realism and evolutionary theory, may offer explanations as to the positive outcome of a negative event, as described in this book.

DEPRESSIVE REALISM

In the early 1970s, experimental psychologist Martin Seligman published research regarding learned helplessness in the face of extreme adversity, suggesting that depression may result from a perceived lack of control over the outcome of an uncontrollable situation, such as trauma:

Not only do we face events that we can control by our actions, but we also face many events about which we can do nothing at all. Such uncontrollable events can significantly debilitate organism: they produce passivity in the face of trauma, inability to learn that responding is effective, and emotional stress in animals, and possibly depression in man (Seligman, 1975, p. 7050).

Shortly after the publication of Seligman's work, Alloy and Abramson (1979) further challenged conventional clinical views of depression by suggesting that, "not only do depressed individuals make realistic inferences but that they do so to a greater extent than non-depressed individuals" (as cited in Moore & Fresco, 2007, p. 144). This theory, depressive realism, stemmed from early studies demonstrating that depressed individuals have better judgment regarding the outcome of their actions, as opposed to non-depressed individuals. In this research, it was found that non-depressed individuals experienced "an illusion of control, in which they consistently overestimated their degree of control over the outcome . . . Depressed individuals experienced no such bias" (Moore & Fresco, 2007, p. 145).

So did the women in this book experience depressive realism? The research itself was not inquiring as to the judgment of contingent events, but the experience of the events as transformative. To date, there have been no studies regarding PPD as an adaptation of depressive realism. While women in this study described enhanced empathy, compassion, and more realistic inferences regarding their needs and potentials, depressive realism does not explain the nature of the growth because of the experience of depression.

Future comparison between transformative PPD and the mechanisms of depressive realism may be fruitful, particularly because women who develop PPD are unique in that they are mothers traditionally given the primary role of caretaking an infant while experiencing depression. Furthermore, for women who experience PPD as a traumatic life event, depressive realism extends the theoretical discussion, but not the practical application of how that event might produce transformative growth or personal development.

What other theories consider the potential growth associated with depression that could explain the growth described in this book? Not surprisingly, anthropology and evolutionary science have examined the role of depressive behavior in human development.

EVOLUTIONARY THEORY

With its stated philosophical roots in the Greek philosophy of Hedonism (Katz, 2013; Moore, 2008), and its legacy noted in the work of Darwin (1872), Lewis (1934), and Bowlby (1980), evolutionary theories of depression propose an interpretation of the depressive symptoms as adaptations to adversity (Hagen, 2011; Hammen, 2005). According to evolutionary anthropologist Edward Hagen, depression can be explained as an adaptation to adversity because it provides benefits to the people experience it (2011).

Evolutionary theory, for the most part, theorizes malignant sadness as psychic pain or distress as a motivator for adaptive response (Hagen, 2011; Tennants, 2002; Trevathan, 2010). From this perspective, PPD might be viewed as maladaptive sadness formed as an affect adaptation to adversity that serves to recover important connections between mother and child, or mother, child, and environment. The "malignant sadness" of PPD serves to repair something broken in the vital connection between this primary and crucial dyad.

Other evolutionary hypotheses, such as social-competition theory and social-risk theory, have proposed somewhat similar theories about the adaptive function of depression (Price et al., 1994). The social-competition theory of evolution determined that depression was an emotion of submission manifested to function to note rank in dominance hierarchies (Price et al., 2007). Social-risk theorists Allens and Badcock (2003) suggested that:

Depressed states evolved to minimize risk in social interactions in which individuals perceive that the ratio of their social value to others, and their social burden on others, is at a critically low level. When this ratio reaches a point where social value and social burden are approaching equivalence, the individual is in danger of exclusion from social contexts that, over the course of evolution, have been critical to fitness (p. 887).

Within social-risk theory, depression serves to reduce threat by increasing sensitivity to signals of others that may threaten them, and by "inhibiting risk-seeking (e.g., confident, acquisitive) behaviors" (Allens & Badcock, 2003, p. 887). Analytical rumination hypothesis (Andrews & Thompson, 2009) proposed that low mood and sadness are responses to social adversity, and serve to trigger psychobiological and neurological responses, which, in turn, signal the individuals to solve complex problems; a trade-off of one impairment for more adaptive impairment results. A common analogy made by Andrews and Thompson (2009) has been that depression is like a fever in this way.

Stress response mechanisms can produce impairments when making trade-offs between different body systems to respond to a stressor. For instance, fever is metabolically expensive and causes significant impairment in multiple domains (work, sexual functioning, social relations, etc.), but these impairments are not usually the product of biological dysfunction. Rather, fever is an adaptation that evolved to coordinate aspects of the immune system in response to infection (p. 621).

From this perspective, could PPD be defined as an "evolved stress mechanism," through which a woman experiences changes in body systems that "promote rumination, the evolved function of which is to analyze the triggering problem" (Andrews & Thompson, 2009, p. 622)? While this variation of evolutionary theory may foster a future understanding of the psychobiological properties and mechanisms of PPD in order to promote problem-solving skills through rumination, this hypothesis does not explain how the symptoms themselves create the conditions for profound personal growth (Hagen, 2011).

POSTTRAUMATIC THEORIES

I was about one year into my data analysis when I had exhausted theoretical literature on depressive realism and evolutionary theories. I knew that based on all the data that I was looking at an experience of trauma.

Could untreated PPD cause psychological trauma? Can PPD itself constitute a trauma? Women are exposed to a life-threatening event: PPD. They are horrified and terrorized by intrusive thoughts, hypervigilance, insomnia, irritability, and physical discomfort, negatively impacting their ability to care for self and others every single day. Moreover, the lack of sleep expands the window of suffering tonight. Without proper intervention, women get no relief from symptoms and no relief from the distress about the symptoms.

Trauma psychology has been examining the ways individuals respond to traumatic life events for decades (Figley, 1978; Horowitz, 1976). The advancements in the field of positive psychology (Linley & Joseph, 2004; Seligman & Csikszentmihalyi, 2000; Snyder & Lopez, 2002) have generated greater theoretical understanding as to the positive emotional states associated with psychological wellbeing. As our understanding of the responses to traumatic events has evolved, we learned that a fundamental response often includes profound personal growth.

POSTTRAUMATIC GROWTH

Tedeschi and Calhoun (2004) defined posttraumatic growth (PTG) in this way: "The term posttraumatic growth refers to positive psychological change experienced as a result of the struggle with highly challenging life circumstances" (p. 1). Expanding the definition of trauma beyond the set criteria of the APA (2000), Tedeschi and Calhoun sought to "describe sets of circumstances that represent significant challenges to the adaptive resources of the individual, and that represent significant challenges to individuals' ways of understanding the world and their place in it" (2004, p. 1). From this theoretical perspective, the experience of PPD described in my research could be defined as a traumatic life event.

PTG theory further extends concepts of recovery, resilience, and survival to include the nature of human beings as growth based. We don't merely recover to pre-trauma levels of functioning. We grow. Our development post-trauma has momentum. Tedeschi and Calhoun explained:

> *Posttraumatic growth describes the experience of individuals whose development, at least in some areas, has surpassed what was present before the struggle with crises occurred. The individual has not only survived but has experienced changes that are viewed as important, and that go beyond what was the previous status quo. Post-traumatic growth is not simply a return to baseline—it is an experience of improvement that for some persons is deeply profound.* (2004, p. 4)

Tedeschi and Calhoun (2004) determined that the term post-traumatic growth best captures the phenomenon for several reasons. According to the authors, the term "stress-related growth" (Tedeschi & Calhoun, 2004, p. 4), used by other growth theories emphasize the nature of the stressful event and minimized the growth potential. Terms that suggested illusory dimensions of transformative change through traumatic life events minimize the ontological reality of transformation. Tedeschi and Calhoun (2004) explained: "In contrast to the terms that emphasize the 'illusions' of people who report these changes, there do appear to be vertical transformative life changes that go beyond illusion" (p. 4).

The quality of the growth experienced by women in this research was beyond the illusion of stress-related growth, demonstrated by the high number of changes of vocation and occupation. The growth described was not explained as a coping mechanism. Significantly, women did not describe thriving or flourishing regarding their perceptions of the transformation. The change experienced was not expressed in rebuilding the old self, nor was it described as changing depression. Depression created the causes for one of life's essential challenges: building a new self with information and wisdom gained through the loss of the old self.

WAS THIS POSTTRAUMATIC GROWTH?

It has been reported that somewhere between 30% and 70% of survivors of traumatic events experienced positive change in some form in their lives (Linley & Joseph, 2004). While the impact of the stressor is negative, the manifestation of the suffering in relation to the stressor is not universal. As I got more clarity that the findings in my study were reflective of posttraumatic growth, a lingering question remained: did the women in my study experience posttraumatic growth?

I corresponded with the authors of the Posttraumatic Growth Inventory (PTGI) and received their permission to use the inventory to perform a posttest with my original sample (N = 20). The PTGI is a 21-item self-report inventory that measures the "extent to which individuals believe they have grown positively from the struggle with the traumatic experience" (Triplett et al., 2012, p. 401).

Five subscales of the PTGI include (a) relating to others, (b) new possibilities, (c) personal strength, (d) spiritual change, and (e) appreciation of life (Tedeschi & Calhoun, 1996). Responses are a 6-point Likert-type scale ranging from 0 (no change) to 5 (great change). Total score (0-105) represents a measurement of posttraumatic growth in the amount, degree, level, extent, and number of benefits (Tedeschi & Calhoun, 1996).

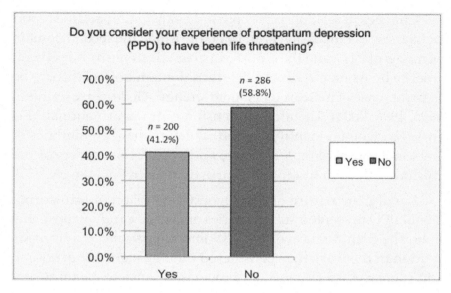

Do you consider your experience of postpartum depression (PPD) to have been life threatening?

Table 1: Posttraumatic Growth Domains and Transformational Dimensions of PPD

I went back to the original sample of women (N = 20) and asked them to complete the Posttraumatic Growth Inventory (PTGI) (Tedeschi & Calhoun, 1996). Each agreed, and with the full sample responding, I was able to determine whether the group, on average, had experienced posttraumatic growth. The average total score was high, 74.8. On average, the women in my sample experienced posttraumatic growth following PPD, demonstrating a theoretical connection supporting untreated PPD as a trauma, and transformation as posttraumatic growth (see Table 1).

From the findings studying the five domains of PTG, appreciation for life was accompanied by a "radically changed sense of priorities" (Tedeschi & Calhoun, 2004, p. 6) that included appreciation for things formerly taken for granted. As noted in the responses, women reprioritizing self-care behaviors after PPD confirmed the first domain of PTG.

Changes in relationships, both losses and gains, and the report of increased compassion after PPD confirmed the second domain of model of PTG, and the report of increased strength and self-confidence by women reflected the third domain of PTG theory, the general sense of increased personal strength (Tedeschi & Calhoun, 1995, 1996, 2004). The after dimension of transformational PPD involved women-identifying and achieving new possibilities in personal, professional, creative, and vocational aspects of life, mirroring the dynamic of the fourth domain in PTG theory.

Finally, the nature of the beyond dimension of transformational PPD presented subcategories of paradox and purpose that echo the fifth domain of PTG. Women experienced a transformation in the ways they considered their existential purpose in life, increased spirituality, and increased sense of meaning and purpose for their experience of PPD.

The experience extended to women beyond recovery, beyond returning to previous levels of psychological well-being, and encompassed the development of wider aspects of self-development, connection to others, sense of purpose, and existential wonder.

CONCLUSION

To date, there is no other research describing untreated postpartum depression as traumatic with the potential for traumatic growth or transformation. As such, I wanted to offer readers critical insight from other experts. And as you will see, I included both agreements and disagreements. Whom do you choose? I charted out the prominent features of my work and asked the experts in each of the areas if they would be so kind as to read my synopsis and tell me what they thought. I knew I needed an expert in trauma and the perinatal period, an expert in posttraumatic growth, an expert in clinical practice, and an expert in postpartum support and advocacy.

CHAPTER 8

PROFESSIONAL PERSPECTIVES

Researchers have focused in on the actual experience
of postpartum depression and not the recovery.
So, I think it's an excellent point that you bring up.
And that's an area that needs to be researched, and
certainly, that would lend to posttraumatic growth.
– Cheryl Beck, personal communication –

As I rounded the corner on writing this book, it occurred to me that while I had attempted to gather a full range of perspectives, I had yet to ask experts for their input on my findings. Why is this important? From a researcher's standpoint, it is essential to get peer review. Handing over your findings for critique is scary, but essential to the establishment of good research.

I spoke with Cheryl Tatano Beck, DNSc, CNM, FAAN about my findings and her thoughts regarding trauma, research, and postpartum depression. I then interviewed a leader in the field of posttraumatic growth, Dr. Jane Shakespeare-Finch, to investigate the validity of my study and gain deeper understanding of PTG theory as it relates to PPD. Next, I interviewed Karen Kleiman, MSW, LCSW—one of the leading clinicians and authors in the field of postpartum mood and anxiety disorders. For this second edition, I have added the perspective of the leading expert in perinatal and mood disorder psychoeducation, Pec Indman, PA, EdD, MFT, PMH-C, EdD.

Cheryl Tatano Beck, DNSc, CNM, FAAN: *"Everything are Data"*

Dr. Cheryl Beck is a Distinguished Professor at the University of Connecticut, School of Nursing. She also has a joint appointment in the Department of Obstetrics and Gynecology at the School of Medicine. Cheryl is a certified nurse-midwife who received her certificate in nurse-midwifery from Yale University. Her Doctor of Nursing Science degree is from Boston University. She is a fellow in the American Academy of Nursing and has received numerous awards such as the Association of Women's Health, Obstetric, and Neonatal Nursing's Distinguished Professional Service Award, Eastern Nursing Research Society's Distinguished Researcher Award, the Distinguished Alumna Award from Yale University, and the Connecticut Nurses' Association's Diamond Jubilee Award for her contribution to nursing research.

Over the past 30 years, Cheryl has focused on developing a research program on postpartum mood and anxiety disorders. Based on the findings from her series of qualitative studies, Cheryl developed the Postpartum Depression Screening Scale (PDSS), which is published by Western Psychological Services.

Cheryl is co-author, with Dr. Denise Polit, of the textbook, *Nursing Research: Generating and Assessing Evidence for Nursing Practice.* Editions of this text received the 2007, 2011, and 2013 American Journal of Nursing Book of the Year Award. Cheryl co-authored, with Dr. Jeanne Driscoll, *Postpartum Mood and Anxiety Disorders: A Clinician's Guide,* which received the 2006 American Journal of Nursing Book of the Year Award. Cheryl's latest two books include *Traumatic Childbirth* and *The Routledge International Handbook of Qualitative Nursing Research.*

The Interview

During the first part of our conversation, I asked Cheryl about the relationship between PPD and trauma. Cheryl has inspired my own interest in research in countless ways. When I had the pleasure of interviewing Cheryl years ago, I asked her how someone knows they are a researcher, and she told me that when you wake up in the morning wondering about your research, you are a researcher. Cheryl's work identifies the gap in research regarding PPD and recovery with a researcher's curiosity, and her wonder as to the fullest possible range of experience for perinatal women, including posttraumatic growth, was affirming as I approached interviewing an expert in posttraumatic growth for feedback on my research.

Walker: Can postpartum depression be traumatic?

Cheryl Beck: Well, from the research I've done and listening to countless women in interviews, I do believe that the moderate-to-severe postpartum depression certainly could be viewed by some women as traumatic, not the mild, and I don't necessarily know those women, but ones that are really struggling with the postpartum depression, so I say moderate-to-severe. If you wanted to classify as traumatic, it would be then at that far-right end, going from mild-to-severe, the women who have severe postpartum depression.

You know, I hadn't asked women in those studies if they perceived their depression as traumatic. It certainly was very difficult time for them, and they struggled. I never asked them about it being perceived as traumatic like I have with the women with their birth process. But I would say some of them would have, probably not all of them would have said it was a traumatic experience if we're looking at traumatic experiences as being horrified about something, fearing for your life. So, I would say some, but not all, women with postpartum depression would view it as that.

You know, many of the women in my studies talked about their loss of self. They didn't know who they were anymore. They were really afraid they would never get their old self back again. Now, I never researched women with postpartum depression viewing it as posttraumatic growth. So, I haven't talked about that, but certainly, they were very fearful that they would never be back to their old selves again, let alone be at a higher place than they were before their depression.

Walker: I'm wondering, is it that we just need to do more research on recovery? We've got so much data about the pathology, what value is there in looking at how women recover, and the nature of that recovery from PPD?

Cheryl Beck: I think you're on an excellent point. You know I have my "Teetering on the Edge" theory (Beck, 1993). I've modified it twice because Glaser [grounded theory research methodologist] always says that everything is data and that your grounded theory shouldn't be stagnant as new research studies are done, or if you collect more data yourself. You constantly are revising.

So, the two revisions that I've done on that theory looked at qualitative studies that had been published since I had done my original grounded theory, which was all done with white, middle-class women. So, when I looked for more qualitative studies published among other cultures to expand my theory, I could ask, what parts of the theory did women from other cultures endorse? Were there some new things?

It was very interesting because the least bit of research has been done on the last phase of my Teetering on the Edge theory, the recovery phase. Really, researchers have focused in on the actual experience of postpartum depression and not the recovery. I think it's an excellent point that you bring up, and that's an area that needs to be researched, and certainly, that would lend to posttraumatic growth.

Jane Shakespeare-Finch, PhD: *"We Need to Normalize the Experience"*

Dr. Jane Shakespeare-Finch is an Associate Professor in the School of Psychology and Counselling at Queensland University of Technology, where she teaches a variety of topics including health psychology, individual differences, and assessment. Jane has enjoyed supervising nearly 50 post-graduate student research projects, including the completed supervision of eight PhD candidates.

Jane's primary area of research is in posttraumatic growth. Starting with emergency service personnel, Jane continues to work with paramedics and police in the promotion of positive post-trauma outcomes and has also investigated the construction of trauma, and post-trauma adaptation and growth in various populations, including refugees and survivors of sexual assault, cancer, and bereavement.

Jane has served as Secretary of the Australasian Society for Traumatic Stress Studies, a member of the International Society for Traumatic Stress Studies and is an international affiliate of the American Psychological Association's trauma division. Jane has published seven books, 13 book chapters, and more than 70 peer-reviewed journal articles and is a regular presenter at national and international conferences. After sending Jane my research to review, we spoke by phone. Our conversation began with her views on the research.

The Interview

Walker: What are your thoughts on the research I presented regarding PPD as a traumatic life event?

Jane Shakespeare-Finch: One of the things that I noticed that you found and that we have found is this notion of increased compassion for other people. That real development of empathy and compassion toward other people, which seems to be kind of a normal thing for many people who've experienced trauma and come out the other end, to want to actually be instrumentally useful to other people.

I think one of the things about your area of research is that society tells us that having a baby is a wonderful thing. And that nurturing comes naturally, you know, like latching on for breastfeeding, it's a natural thing, but for many women, that simply is not the reality. So you then have these expectations of everything going well, the birth going well, the baby being beautiful and having all the things it's meant to have, and then happy families going home and looking after babies and moving forward, whereas in actual fact, it completely, fundamentally shifts who you are as a person.

And when that event doesn't work the way you expected it to, there's much self-doubt and self-blame for things not working the way that the books have told you or society has told you it will. And I see that could quite easily lead to a spiral of downward effect, etc., as one beats themselves up that they don't look like the celebrities on the TV, and they're not shedding all their kilos and looking wonderful and feeling just dynamic about being a new mom.

One of the things we may fail to do in a therapeutic setting is to draw on people's strengths, to recognize them, and reflect them back. We have to normalize the experience that people are having. We've been doing quite a lot of work with sexual assault survivors recently, and the same thing is happening there. This is devastating, yes, it is, but most women who have experienced childhood sexual assault do go on to be fully functioning adults—the way in which we intervene can have a lot to do with that.

Walker: What would you see as some of the gross misunder-standings about posttraumatic growth?

Jane Shakespeare-Finch: I think one of the first things that springs to mind is this argument in the literature that post-traumatic growth is illusionary. That it's the positive spin people put on things to help them cope with an experience. And that's a fundamental misunderstanding about the way in which people actually do truly transform their lives as a result of that struggle that they engage in. I think that's one of the fundamental problems.

The other is confusion between what is growth and what is resilience, which is only just recently getting a bit of air. But when you have people who are prolific in the literature sort of saying, "No, this doesn't exist. This is some sort of artifi-cial illusionary coping strategy," then it makes it difficult for those of us who actually sit there with people who've survived trauma to be heard.

The other difference, I think, between posttraumatic growth, and some of the other concepts like thriving, flourishing, and stress-related growth is that in Richard [Tedeschi] and Lawrence's [Calhoun] model, and you've found it in your research, is that the experience has to be one that shatters your previous assumptions about the world, about your place in the world, about the predictability and safety of the world, about good things happening to good people and bad things happening only to bad people, that kind of thing if you can use those dichotomies.

And so, I think the fact that the posttraumatic growth model is solidly embedded in cognitive theory and requires that schematic shattering in order to rebuild your sense of who you are in the world and incorporate or weave that experience into your life, makes it different to some of the other concepts.

Walker: How do you see posttraumatic growth as a component of care for clinicians?

Jane Shakespeare-Finch: I think the posttraumatic growth model is the most comprehensive and sensible model that we have to look at positive post-trauma life changes. And there is very little recognition of the fact that, for many people, the experience that can provide the catalyst for symptoms of PTSD is the same experience that provides the catalyst for growth. And these things can and do co-occur.

A psychologist's job is to sort of disentangle psychological disorder, correctly identify a diagnosis and formulate some sort of intervention whereas, I actually think a solution-based approach to trauma research and to practice is much more beneficial for the people that you're aiming to help. And this model that Richard [Tedeschi] and Lawrence [Calhoun] came up with didn't come out of thin air. It was created over 20 years, as working clinicians, as well as academics, and seeing the real changes that were made, especially in the lives of bereaved parents.

One of the things that we always need to say right up front is that people finding a positive transformation through their experiences does not, for a second, deny the very devastating experiences that they had in the first instance. And that it doesn't mean that this is one outcome as opposed to another outcome, that there are interplays of many outcomes for people.

As I was saying before about having a good day, but that doesn't mean that you might not hear a piece of music or see something that reminds you of a time when you were in the depths of despair and that it's perfectly all right to allow yourself to feel those emotions. Not everything in life is wonderful and glossy, and you don't want to sell posttraumatic growth as something that can be perceived to be illusionary, because it's not.

I think having really practical ways of trying to express to people that yes, you've got research that backs up what you have found here, but these are the real ways in which people, allied health professionals and people who are surviving these experiences, can engage with themselves, with their thought process, with their emotions, with their relationships with other people, to create a new narrative that isn't laden with that, "Hang on a second, this isn't the way life is supposed to be, therefore, somehow, I have failed." And that beating up of self that happens. I think we just need to be much more honest about the human condition and speak in terms that are accessible to people.

Dr. Shakespeare-Finch offers a critical review of clinical implications for posttraumatic growth interventions. What struck me in speaking with her was her acknowledgment of the human condition as both flawed and filled with possibility. Underlying current research we have regarding the pathology of PPD, lays a sensible, pragmatic, solution-based belief—of course, women grow through suffering. The concept of growth through PPD as viewed as a traumatic life event, isn't as much new as it is not articulated by research and theoretical literature, such as depressive realism and evolutionary theory.

Secondly, women grow *through* suffering. As noted, growth through adversity is well documented in philosophical, psychological, and religious literatures. Traditional science and epistemologies of science have examined growth through adversity as well. From Aristotle's eudaimonism to Carl Roger's organismic growth theory, Maslow, Rollo May, Laszlo, positive psychology, and now posttraumatic growth have examined growth through adversity as an integral component of the human condition.

What has *not* been made as obvious, however, is the identification of PPD as one of those adversities. We don't call PPD traumatic. As providers and researchers, how we disentangle the seeming conflicting ontologies of growth and suffering is critical to our ability to recognize growth potential in the face of adversity for women who experience PPD. As I learned from my interview with Karen Kleiman, disentangling the language of suffering itself can be problematic.

Karen Kleiman, MSW, LCSW:
"Is it a Big T or a little t?"

Karen Kleiman, MSW, LCSW, is well-known as an international expert on postpartum depression and anxiety, and advocate for perinatal women and their families. Her work has been featured online and within the mental health community for three decades. In 1988, Karen founded *The Postpartum Stress Center*, a premier treatment and training facility for prenatal and postpartum depression and anxiety disorders, where she treats individuals and couples.

More recently, she founded The Postpartum Stress & Family Wellness Center in New Jersey. Karen is featured as an expert on PsychologyToday.com as a "Best Voice in Psychology," and is the author of her blog, *This Isn't What I Expected: Notes on Healing Postpartum Depression*.

In addition to her clinical work at The Postpartum Stress Center, she created and instructs a professional training course for clinicians who have an interest in specializing in the treatment of postpartum distress. Karen is the author of several top-selling books on postpartum depression. Her first book, *This Isn't What I Expected: Overcoming Postpartum Depression* co-authored with Valerie Davis Raskin, forged new territory in the self-help book market on postpartum depression. Karen's book has proven to be an essential resource for women and their families.

The Interview

I interviewed Karen specifically for her feedback as a clinician with unparalleled expertise in treating PPD. How does she view my findings within her own experience? Were there elements of care provider failure that resonated with her experience? What would she make of the theory that PPD can be experienced as a traumatic life event? What is shared here are the segments of our conversation regarding (a) care providers, (b) suicidality, and (c) PPD as trauma. Karen's insights provided invaluable feedback and begged further discussion.

I explained to Karen the high level of care provider failure reported in my research. Karen described her understanding of the compartmentalization of physical and mental illness by care providers.

Karen Kleiman: Postpartum depression symptoms are the feelings that a woman has are expressed as symptoms, but they are experienced as self. So, we say, when somebody is sick, and she goes to the doctor, and she has a sore throat, and she has swollen glands, and it hurts to swallow, and she has a fever. The doctor says, "Oh, here's a cluster of symptoms. I know what this is. And I know how to treat it."

And when a woman has postpartum depression, she says to us, "I'm a bad mother; I am powerless over how I am feeling. I will always feel this way. My loved ones will abandon me." And when I, as the clinician, hear those sentences, "she thinks she's a terrible person," I hear she has a sore throat, and she has a fever. Right? I say to women all the time, that this is not about you. This is about your symptoms. These are symptoms. When you get better, you will no longer feel this way.

Symptoms became a theme of our conversation. I shared the high levels of suicidality ideation in my research and asked for her reflections.

Karen Kleiman: I think we have no idea how big suicidal ideation is. And what I always say is if you don't ask every single postpartum woman if she's having thoughts of suicide, you have no freaking idea. And these are women *that look* like you and me and are going to their doctors, and they're asked how they're feeling, and they're saying they're fine, and they're going home thinking of ways to kill themselves.

Luckily, the numbers aren't as high as the symptoms are, but I think that the disparity that women are faced with, with motherhood, within the context of being a mother feeling this way, mental illness aside, mental illness alone is bad enough, but you stick a baby in there? "My baby would be way better off without me." I mean, hello. You don't have to look very far to feel that way. So, think that thoughts of suicide, I think that people are missing that all over the place. And fortunately, a lot of these women are just getting better. They're just getting better. But I think a lot of clinicians are looking at these women that look really good, and look really healthy, are not asking them how many glasses of wine they're having a night.

Karen's insights as to the symptoms associated with suicidal ideation in PPD are chilling and merit attention. How might the experience of suicidal ideation relate to a direct experience of trauma? If trauma involves exposure to a life-threatening event, wouldn't suicidal ideation during untreated PPD be traumatic?

The conversation with Karen regarding PPD as trauma continued to provide thought-provoking questions as to how we unpack symptoms and understand a woman's experience of those symptoms relative to the diagnostic criteria. In asking Karen about clients experiencing PPD as a trauma, she shared the following:

Karen Kleiman: It's interesting as I was thinking about this in preparation to talk to you. I was seeing that my population is really split down the middle. It feels like half the women that I see, and this is just anecdotal, obviously—half the women that I see sort of take this what I'm going use your word "trauma," even with the little small t, and not a big T. And they take this trauma, and they carry it with them as if they continue to be burdened by it forever. And they are angry, and they are tired, and they are frustrated, and their marriage is impaired, and they literally cannot move forward or let go, which is what I see is one of my greatest challenges is to help them learn that.

The other half and these are just women who stay in treatment, obviously, so I'm not seeing the women that get better and leave. But the other half of the women that stay are women who are falling more into the category that you're describing, who feel that maybe something good has come out of it, maybe my marriage has strengthened, maybe awareness is more acute, maybe my ability to take care of myself has been initiated through this process.

And sure, I mean, we hear things like that all the time. I wouldn't wish this on my worst enemy, but I've grown into a better person because of it. And so, then we know that in terms of the trauma literature that the same two people can be in the same trauma, and one of them is paralyzed by anxiety or incapacitated by their trauma. And the other one goes on to teach about it, and write about it, and save the world because of it.

So, the resilience in terms of who they are is also very relevant. I have to tell you that that's one of the things that we do in therapy is talk about sort of the characteristics that are associated with that kind of positive adaptation. You know what I mean? And when I see somebody struggling, one of the things that we do, not right away, but as she's healing, is we take, literally, a list of the characteristics. Like the ability to plan, and seek support, and find humor, and insight, and all this stuff. And we go through it, and I say to her, "If you're not good at these things, let's work on these things. These are the characteristics that are associated with a better recovery and a positive adaptation of this trauma, so to speak."

As a clinician, Karen integrates appreciation for a woman's ability to adapt to PPD in positive ways. Through her clinical interview and establishing therapeutic rapport, Karen encourages her clients to acknowledge characteristic strengths and weaknesses in order to facilitate and promote growth and recovery. But what of the traumatic impact of PPD?

Karen Kleiman: But that is sort of what gets me confused. The word "trauma" actually gets me confused. That's the part that I'm not sure I can articulate. I'm not sure I see this in the same way in terms of PTSD and that. I see it as something that I can't really define yet, which I probably should have done before I talked to you. But I see it as sort of the breaking down of the soul and devastation in mind, in spirit is not something to me as a trauma.

It's traumatic, but in terms of the definition of a trauma, I just don't see it as PTSD. I just don't see it. Now, is it there, and I'm not seeing it or what's happening? But I don't see it in my practice. And trust me, I'm looking for it.

I see this other thing. I see a loss of confidence, and I see sort of the breakdown of who I used to be, and how do I get that back, and sort of that dream that I was describing, that my insides were all over the place. So, I don't see that. Clearly, that's traumatic, and we're probably both saying the same thing, but the word "trauma," in its clinical sense, doesn't always apply to what I'm saying.

Part of the wonderful experience of interviewing Karen is her willingness to critically unpack ideas while infusing her own expertise. She holds her space as an expert clinician and invites dialogue that may or may not lead to mutual agreement. These are the conversations that challenge us to grow: reflect on what we know, review what we want to know, and reframe our paradigm.

What she offers here is an invaluable reflection for care providers, scholars, and women. We need to question the medical language used to label disorder. Clinicians should not be confused by reconciling the perception of a client's experience with a diagnostic label.

From Karen's perspective, one can understand how clinicians might struggle to align PPD with trauma, given the limited language of the diagnostic manual. The criteria, defined by medical science, must match the condition presented by the client in order to signify the disorder noted in the manual.

Another example of disconnect in diagnostic criteria for women during the childbearing period is apparent in the absence of postpartum onset criteria for trauma disorders. There are no postpartum or perinatal-onset specifier for trauma disorders, despite substantive research identifying traumatic childbirth.

Think about this for a moment. There is a plethora of research on "traumatic childbirth," yet no diagnostic criteria in the medical manuals to diagnose "traumatic childbirth" or PTSD related to childbirth. A woman may experience hours of invasive medical procedures done to her genitals (episiotomy, forceps, vacuum extraction, intrauterine catheter, artificial rupture of amniotic membranes, countless cervical checks, Foley/urine catheter), witness the loss of blood (postpartum hemorrhage), had to have blood infusions, been told that the life of her child is in danger while hospital protocol mandates constant external fetal monitoring (audible heart rate of the baby), been confined to bed and not allowed to eat or drink for the duration of labor and birth—or worse, a medical emergency for herself or her baby (as if none of what was listed before this wasn't tantamount to an emergency).

If that woman develops symptoms of distress relative to the childbirth that impairs her ability to care for herself or her infant, what diagnosis does she receive? There is none. If she presents her symptoms to a medical care provider, be it in the OB/GYN's office or emergency room, the default diagnosis would be postpartum depression or anxiety. The treatment protocol would be for PPD/PPA, not PTSD. The medication, therapy, and care would be for PPD/PPA, not PTSD.

How do these practices happen? Providers have taught them. Systems of education teach professionals to use specific words for the symptoms they see. Textbooks define the terms. Students are tested their knowledge of the term and accurate application to cases. Institutions of learning and accrediting bodies confer student's ability to use these words, and off they go, licensed to practice using these words as ways of helping. What, in turn, ends up happening is that it becomes the client or patient's responsibility to describe their symptoms in a manner that matches the medical manual definition.

Consider a hypothetical OB/GYN. Technically, her profession is that of a surgeon, but nonetheless, she has been given the responsibility of detecting symptoms of PPD and referring to appropriate care providers or treating the symptoms herself. She completed a four-year residency, during which she had one six-week rotation in psychiatry. Before that, she attended medical school where she spent four years studying biology, physiology, anatomy, and chemistry. Before that, she attended high school, where the required curriculum included; biology, physiology, anatomy, and chemistry for four years. She may have been able to take art, music, and sports as well. Before that, she attended elementary and middle school, where the core curriculum included biology, physiology, anatomy, and chemistry.

So, on this day, a perfectly well-meaning, highly trained woman looks at another woman. They look at one another through the thick lens of nearly 25 years of education on biology, physiology, anatomy, and chemistry. The reality created is that one woman is a doctor, one woman is a patient. One is well, one is potentially sick. They have come together that day for the doctor to assess the normal from the abnormal symptoms of the patient, based on the biology, physiology, anatomy, and chemistry taught to her for 25 years.

Yet, despite all of the knowledge and training, the practice of evidence-based medicine, and diagnostic criteria, the doctor only sees pathology because she's only been trained to use one tool: science. And still, doctors get it wrong. How we educate our providers deserves relentless review, which is why I have added an interview with the leading international PPD/PPA educator, Pec Indman.

Pec Indman, PA, EdD, MFT, PMH-C, EdD: *"I Think It IS a Big T for Many Women"*

For 27 years, Pec worked as a psychotherapist specializing in perinatal mental health. She's a former family practice trained Physician Assistant and has a master's degree in health psychology and a doctorate in counseling. She became one the first psychotherapists in the country to earn national certification in Perinatal Mental Health. Pec has been creating curriculum and training nationally and internationally for Postpartum Support International since 1999. She has served on the PSI board of directors as the Chair of Education and Training, and currently serves on the PSI Advisory Council. An invited speaker, Pec has trained for WIC programs, multiple hospital Grand Rounds, county public health departments, the Health Resources & Services Administration (Adolescent and Child Health Bureau), breastfeeding coalitions, and many other organizations.

She's contributed to the American College of OB/GYN Maternal Mental Health Bundle, articles for the *Journal of Obstetric, Gynecologic & Neonatal Nursing* and the *Journal of Perinatology*. She is the co-author of the award-winning book *Beyond the Blues, Understanding and Treating Prenatal and Postpartum Depression & Anxiety* (2019).

The Interview

Walker: What do you think happens when a woman is symptomatic, and providers don't recognize it? What is the disconnect?

Pec: Well, I think if you're not looking for it or asking the questions, you're not going to find it. We have a slide in the PSI training that shows women who were diagnosed by a provider versus women who were screened, the same women, and most of the providers totally missed it because they didn't ask.

We did a survey in the Mountain View area near Silicon Valley before the outpatient maternal mental health program got started and asked providers if they screened for perinatal mood and anxiety disorders. And I was shocked at how many said they did screen. I wonder what . . . Were they actually, you know, pen and paper screening, or were they saying, "How are you doing?" And that in their mind was screening

Providers aren't trained to screen. You know, it's the whole issue of time, it's the issue of they don't necessarily have a referral or know where to send them. Will they get reimbursed for screening? They tend not to be trained in how to rule out bipolar disorder, which is often misdiagnosed as unipolar depression.

When I was in San Jose, there was a large group of OB/GYNs who would often refer women to me for psychotherapy. Women would come into their office, and the providers would ask some questions, and then they were very happy to hand them a prescription for Zoloft and say, you know, "We really encourage you go see Pec for psychotherapy." And they'd give them my card.

The women were anxious about the medication because nobody had really talked to them about it. I'd do a thorough screening, and often, I'd determine that the woman actually had bipolar disorder. I'd call the doctor back and say, "Hey, you know, this is great. You screened and you provided medications, but it's probably not the right medication. And she needs to see a psychiatrist." And then they would . . . they started handing out antidepressant prescriptions and said, "But don't fill in 'til you talk to Pec." So, I think they don't have training. They don't have the time.

Walker: And they are not mandated to screen.

Pec: They're not mandated. Perinatal providers are not mandated to screen for mental health. ACOG improved their screening recommendations, but they are still quite weak and inadequate. The American Academy of Family Practice and the American Academy of Pediatrics all have recommendations. But there's no mandate. That's a huge challenge.

One of the things I think your book is doing is calling on consumers to be more educated. I think we need to educate families. And we need to educate providers to screen, we need people trained how to treat because as we know, even therapists, most of us have not had any particular training.

I am a Family Practice trained Physician Assistant. My master's degree is in health psychology. My doctorate is in marital and family therapy. There was not one mention of perinatal mental health. So, as a treatment provider, you have to look for specific training, which is unfortunate. It should be a basic part of every medical and psychological training. So, I think we're missing the boat on all three of those, you know, that women and families need to be more educated. That's why Shoshana Bennett and I wrote the book, Beyond the Blues, Understanding and Treating Prenatal and Postpartum Depression and Anxiety.

Walker: I often reflect on the fact that from the moment women know they are pregnant, they interact [with] healthcare providers. Women are screened, asked about our family history of diabetes to look for gestational diabetes, obesity, cancer, hypertension, etc.

But women are not asked about their mental health symptoms or family history. It seems, unfortunately, we still have so far to go to put mental health in the prenatal health screening protocol. Am I on track in that thinking?

Pec: Yes. Women know they're going to have their pee checked for diabetes. They're going to have their weight checked. Their blood pressure is going be checked. Where's the brain?

I had a slide in a presentation, and it had a picture with a doll, but her head was torn off. And it's like, you know, the brain is connected to the body. You can't separate them, and we need to be paying attention to what the brain does because that controls the whole rest of the body.

It makes no sense, and it's bad for our health. If we're concerned about women having good perinatal outcomes, we need to look at the brain. It's connected, and we know the risks of having a perinatal mood and anxiety disorder during pregnancy are not good. It's not benign.

Walker: In the first edition, I asked different professionals if untreated postpartum depression can be experienced as a traumatic life event. It's very interesting to get a different perspective. For example, Karen Kleiman shared that she differentiated between a "big T" a "little t" trauma and that the experience of trauma as a result of untreated PPD is a "little t." What are your thoughts about untreated PPD as a traumatic life event?

Pec: I think it is a big T for many women. As Cheryl Beck says, "Trauma is in the eye of the beholder." I think for so many women, the experience is like you're in a blackhole for a critical time in their lives. Many women don't seek treatment for years or don't get treatment at all. We'll do a training or talk to a group and people will come up and say, "Oh, my God, that's what I had 20 years ago, and I never told a soul. And I suffered with the consequences, my family suffered . . ."

We know that about 19% of perinatal women have thoughts of suicide. That is traumatic. Many women have trauma from psychiatric hospitalizations or having the police or child protective services called. It affected them long term and continues to impact their lives.

As they heal, many feel reborn and stronger. They become a therapist, or they become doula or become an advocate or volunteer or I have a woman who became a competitive weightlifter, you know. She felt powerful! A perinatal mood or anxiety disorder can be really a huge chunk out of somebody's life. It can be lifechanging.

My experience with women is they feel as if they are sucked into this vast, deep hole and it's tenacious. It keeps them there. They're smothering, they're dying, they are scared, helpless, and hopeless. The fear of losing your mind and your life as you knew it—it's horrifying.

In our book, we mentioned a woman who had had cancer prior to her postpartum depression. She said when she had cancer, she was so afraid she would die. When she had postpartum depression, she wanted to die. Frequently, women said, "I can't live another day like this." They feel tortured by the illness and the accompanying guilt and shame. "I am suffering," "I can't keep doing this." And unfortunately, the nature of depression is helpless and hopeless. So, there's no way out and you can't see that when you're really depressed.

Often as women recovered and look back, they recognized their strength and accomplishment of overcoming the monster of perinatal illness. One client I had who was a triathlete said it "kicked her butt" but "If I can recover from this, I can accomplish anything!"

Perinatal mood and anxiety disorders are viewed differently than other disorders in our society. Many people are still unaware that perinatal illness exists or that there are a number of different kinds of effective treatment. And unlike other kinds of illnesses, there is still so much inaccurate information.

Walker: Do you think that there is a way that mental health clinicians might be open to bringing trauma language into perinatal mood and anxiety disorder language? To date, trauma has been used in relation to traumatic childbirth, would clinicians be better informed about looking for signs of trauma as a result of untreated mood disorders?

Pec: Yes. We just put in a section in the PSI training about trauma-informed care because sexual abuse as, you know, a young person impacts perinatal mental health. And there actually was a good recent article in "The Green Journal," the ACOG journal, not too long ago about doing trauma-informed care. You can't take one part of a woman's life or anybody's life out of the context of their history and their past.

One of the ways we can help women with a perinatal mood or anxiety disorders in their healing is to teach them about the language of resilience and talk to them about post-traumatic growth.

Walker: What I see coming across my research feed every day are studies about how maternal mental illness damages *children* across their lifespan. But little to no research is generated about how these illnesses affect *women* across the lifespan. No one is looking at women, nor asking them about their experiences.

Pec: I agree, Walker. I think our society has done a poor job with mental health overall, in all groups and ages. We have more information now than ever about transgenerational trauma. How it's passed from parent to child. So, I think there has been increased access to education for providers in their basic training. There programs that do postdoc programs and are training a few psychiatrists here and there.

But you know, as I mentioned, the ACOG has increased their call for perinatal mental health screening. ACOG has created a maternal mental health safety bundle, in addition to "safety bundles" for things like hemorrhage. Is anybody reading it?

Walker: I'm wondering if you've noticed any changes in how these disorders present themselves. Is anything different? Are you seeing more bipolar? Are you seeing more anxiety? Are there any changes in the actual manifestation of the disease?

Pec: I learned years ago to start asking questions about anxiety, bipolar symptoms of mood elevation and family history, so I found it. I hadn't been asking those questions. As a therapist, I hadn't really learned to ask those questions.

I think I saw more anxiety. I think people were more comfortable talking about that than depression. But I really was aware of the huge comorbidity. Women were anxious about their depression, and depressed about their anxiety, and depressed about intrusive thoughts, and anxious about intrusive thoughts. So, the comorbidity was really for me monumental. I rarely saw someone who just had depression because it's anxiety-producing to be depressed. And, it's depressing and frightening to be anxious.

It's hard for women to separate one from the other, and especially in terms of anxiety involving friends and not wanting people to see you depressed. There's anxiety around what are people going to think about you and your ability to parent.

Walker: Stigma.

Pec: Stigma, yes. And if there's a shame about breastfeeding on top of that? Women feel like they are going to get yelled at for breastfeeding in public or yelled at for bottle feeding in public. People are always telling you what to do and trying to be helpful, and it's not always helpful advice or wanted advice.

Walker: And to jump in on that same idea, if someone gets a cancer diagnosis, cancer is not associated with motherhood. A diagnosis that has been historically and continues to be associated with the idea of good or bad mother carries tremendous stigma.

Pec: Yes. Generally speaking, you don't get blamed for having cancer. No one would ask you or expect you to "snap out of it." But with a "brain illness," there is blame, shame, and guilt. When someone has cancer, family and friends often rally to help with food, transportation, and childcare. With

219

a perinatal illness, there is often a lack of understanding and support.

Walker: Maybe one thing that's changed and can help to address stigma is the language we use. We're at least saying, you know, perinatal mood and anxiety disorders regularly, we've gotten our brains in the habit of saying that. We have changed the letters PPD to PMAD. I think that's a step in the right direction because if we're using words that speak to a broader and more inclusive phenomenon, it's got to be helpful.

Pec: That is a huge advancement because it used to be PPD, postpartum depression, and everything was lumped under that umbrella. People used to believe it was on a linear spectrum of worsening. We're really recognizing there's different illness, and you know, we're talking more about postpartum psychosis. There's more information becoming available about that. So, that is another advancement. I mean, it's just progress is slow.

We've been doing this work for a long time. Progress is slow in coming, like any systemic change. It's got to take a lot of work to make changes. And, we need changes on multiple fronts.

Sadly, there will be more deaths and more suffering before people are going to recognize how critical and important this is and how long-lasting the effects on the women, the family, relationships, and work. I mean, now we're talking about intergenerational trauma and you know, that this continues. We're setting up our young people for depression and chronic mental illness, and we need to put a stop to it.

Jane Honikman, Founder, Postpartum Support International (PSI): As Simple as That

I read *I'm Listening* by Jane Honikman, in 2007. When I received the book, Jane included a hand-written thank you note in the package, a gesture of manners I remember to this day. I met Jane Honikman in person in 2010. I walked into a conference ballroom at the Marce conference in Pittsburgh. I recognized her immediately. She looked at the book in my hand and said, "I LOVE that book!" I was reading the recently released book *Half the Sky: Turning Oppression into Opportunity for Women Worldwide* (Kristof & WuDunn, 2010). We spoke briefly, and I took my seat for the luncheon where Jane was slated to give opening remarks.

I sat listening to Jane's speech, getting angry. Not at her, nor the content, but the clinking of silverware and casual conversations taking place while she spoke. I was there to hear what the woman who had single-handedly built PSI had to say. I learned then that sometimes when strong women speak, we forget our manners. We shouldn't.

Jane developed PSI in the midst of the women's liberation movement in the U.S.—and speaks about feminism from a lived experience that I personally find incredibly important and valuable. Obviously, I went into my interview with Jane, totally biased. That said, I knew that she would offer me the same critical eye and authenticity I had come to admire.

I had interviewed Jane before and have had many conversations with her over the years. Jane pulls no punches, is a pragmatic optimist, and has a mind that is constantly moving to connect people in meaningful ways. She plays the flute, prefers the phone to email, and has met with her closest friends every Tuesday for breakfast for the last 30 years.

When I interviewed Jane for this book, I drove to her home in Santa Barbara. I sat at her kitchen table, watching her hop around her kitchen, loading the dishwasher, and preparing lunch: heirloom tomatoes from her garden, and leftover butternut squash lasagna made by her daughter-in-law, sliced avocado, and crackers. I was used to Jane's straightforward style and wondered what she would have to say about this theory of mine—PPD as trauma and transformation. As usual, her laser-like insight did not disappoint.

In discussing the current state of PPD, I asked Jane about the prevalence rates for PPD remaining the same (or higher) since she began her advocacy work in the 1980s.

Jane: No, the rates haven't changed, and everybody wants them to be worse. And so, they are. That's the other thing that I witnessed over these years. Oh, good grief, as bad enough as it is, just leave it alone and just stay with what are we going to do about it? We need to talk about it and tell women to be open and honest about how you're feeling. And it's not just women; it's men too. Simple as that.

Walker: What about the thought that women experience PPD as traumatic and can grow as a result?

Jane: Well, again, my experience early on was that the people who called me said that very same thing. They said, "It was the worst thing that ever happened to me, but I'm glad I had to go through it, and now I'm going to help others." Walker, we keep going around in circles and talking as if the next person that thinks it up is the first person who's thought if it. I think we just spin. And we don't support women. Simple as that.

Simple as that. Our conversation moved to other subjects that day. I drove home wondering, am I reinventing the wheel?

PROFESSIONAL PERSPECTIVES

I knew that the women's stories of trauma and growth described something different than what had been described about PPD. But maybe I was just adding modifiers to the word postpartum— spinning language without real consequence.

CONCLUSION

Much like my interview with Dr. Shakespeare-Finch, my take-away from Jane's interview was that PPD as a trauma was not as much a discovery as a *rediscovery* of something that has been there all along—women's ability to grow through adversity. The description of the suffering associated with PPD by medical and psychological professionals has remained consistent—that's the spinning. We recycle the same descriptions of symptoms. We circle through evidence regarding prevalence, symptoms, risk factors, and negative outcomes. We spin symptoms—not growth potential.

CHAPTER 9

WHEN PPD GROWS UP: NEW REFLECTIONS AND FUTURE DIRECTIONS

What fabrications they are, mothers. Scarecrows,
wax dolls for us to stick pins into, crude diagrams.
We deny them an existence of their own, we make
them up to suit ourselves—our own hungers,
our own wishes, our own deficiencies.
– Margaret Atwood, *The Blind Assassin* –

By the time I got home from my interview with Jane, I had realized that I had one more transcription to review: Jane's own postpartum diary. Jane had documented her own experience of PPD in her first book, *Step by Step: A Guide to Organizing a Postpartum Parent Support Network in Your Community* (Honikman, 2000). Analyzing her writing might provide final insight into the theory that PPD is traumatic and transformational.

In Chapter 1: "My Postpartum Diary," Jane shares her personal diary of a difficult first pregnancy in the 1960s as an unwed young woman, her extraordinary sadness over giving her daughter up for adoption, and her experiences of postpartum depression and anxiety with her second and third baby years later. Jane's experience of PPD in 1972 echoed the women's voices from this book. Indeed, struggling to survive and transforming through that struggle was Jane's story as well. Following the birth of her son in the spring of 1972, Jane remarked on how unprepared she felt, mirroring the experience of the women in this book (Honikman, 2000):

I'd had an expectation that maternal instinct would wash over me and guide me through each day. It started when we came home from the security and support of the hospital. I put my baby in his cozy bed, stood beside him, and thought, "Now what do I do?"

Jane described the symptoms of depression with falling, downward directional language similar to the women in my research, "From triumph and exhilaration of this birth, I've plunged into this morass of feeling overwhelmed and exhausted, alone, and frightened" (Honikman, 2000, p. 18).

By March of 1972, Jane was struggling with breastfeeding, exhaustion, and increasing symptoms of PPD.

The baby's schedule is like a Ferris wheel in high gear, whirling and spinning. I feel like a damp washcloth being wrung out for the hundredth time as I nurse constantly. When I attended a nursing mother's group and confessed that I've been using supplemental bottles, I could feel their glares of disapproval, not to mention silent disgust. Mom came down for a few days but couldn't or didn't want to stay. I feel incredibly alone. What am I going to do to survive this hideous existence (Honikman, 2000, p. 18)?

And as the symptoms became more severe, Jane experienced care provider failure not unlike the women in this book. Jane's diary entry, from May 1972 described:

The other day I fainted from trying to contain a pain in my chest. The doctor checked me for physical ailments and then sent me home. He never asked how I was feeling emotionally, so I certainly didn't volunteer information about my vast sense of inadequacy, terrible mood swings, poor sleeping, lack of concentration and anxiousness (Honikman, 2000, p. 19).

Sound familiar? Reading this the first time, remembering fainting during my own battle with PPD, I realized that researching was as much about the past as the present and future. I thought about 1972: Jane as a young mother fainting—her fear, frailty, while about 70 miles away. I had just turned 5-years-old, my fainting spell some 30 years in the future. Jane's suffering created the causes for the advent of PSI, and through a web of connections and advocacy, made its way to me, and through me to so many. I realized then, and have learned since, that history has substantive power. History informs us in every moment.

In August of 1972, Jane began to feel relief and shared how support from other mothers was crucial to her getting better.

I've made new friends with other new mothers at a child study group through AAUW. They've helped me realize I'm not crazy or alone. It's a form of therapy, I guess. My stomach aches and head-aches are not as frequent now, probably because I'm sleeping and eating better lately (p. 20).

Following a recurrence of PPD in 1974 after the birth of her daughter, Jane went beyond PPD—finding a purpose for her suffering in helping others. In July of 1977, Jane wrote:

My vow of long ago has finally taken on a form and direction. I have a purpose now beyond being a mother and a wife, with energy coming from that unspoken force in the back of my mind. My friends and I have launched a community-based, grassroots, self-help parent support program. We got funding from a grant from AAUW. It's an idea born from our own experiences and needs. We've named it Postpartum Education for Parents, "PEP" for short, and laughed about not calling the organization "After-birth." The word "postpartum" is not in the public's vocabulary yet, but it is that period of time from birth through the first year of a baby's life (Honikman, 2000, p. 22).

Jane had experienced the same journey in the 1970s as the women in my research in 2014 and now in 2020. She was unprepared, shattered by PPD twice, slowly got better, and then grew beyond recovery. Jane experienced growth beyond being a wife and mother, and an energy coming from an "unspoken force" that fueled new ideas, possibilities, and potential, resulting in the growth of her advocacy work and her innate potential.

For all intents and purposes, one could say that Jane experienced posttraumatic growth as a result of her untreated PPD. And anyone who knows Jane would tell you that she continues to grow as a result of those events to this day. That's one of the messages of this book: untreated PPD can be a traumatic life event that triggers traumatic stress responses, including the potential for posttraumatic growth.

In revising this chapter for the second edition, I realized that I needed to remember something else Jane shared with me in a 2013 interview for Science and Sensibility. In discussing how to make the changes necessary for better treatment and outcomes for PPD, she said, "Honesty is disarming. It should set the stage for dialogue." I can attest to Jane's practice of disarming honesty. Her fearless candor is exactly what is needed to examine how PPD can "grow up."

NEW REFLECTIONS

What are we missing? What frank, honest conversations can we have about this thing we call "PPD?" Looking back on the first edition of this book and considering the current state of PPD in research and advocacy, I am struck by the landscape of research. today is in many ways as it was when I wrote the first edition in 2013, as it was for myself in 2000, as it was for my mother in 1967 and her mother in 1935, as it was for Jane in 1972 and 1974.

We need change. We need fundamental change in the language and ownership of the knowledge regarding women and their experience of the perinatal mood and anxiety disorders over their entire lifespan—not only in the months after birth.

CHANGING LANGUAGE

In her brilliant book, *The Ghost in the House: Real Mothers Talk about Maternal Depression, Raising Children, and How They Cope,* Tracy Thompson described depression in this way:

> . . . *when you are surveying the wreckage of your life—and the exact cause of the devastation at some point ceases to be relevant— the question you must confront is the same one depression poses: How do I live now? The unique nature of depression is that it gets you to that question directly; no external catastrophe is required* (Thompson, 2006, p. 210).

With no observable external event, save the birth of a baby, untreated PPD can strip life down to the barest bones, and beg the biggest questions, such as, how do I live now? This book has shared examples of answers to those questions—as told by women themselves. Their stories are more than novel narratives of outlier moms—women who "survive" and feel a sense of cliché gratitude for the experience. This is not a collection of stories of silver linings.

What the women in this book described, and the experts confirmed, is that untreated PPD is a traumatic life event. Broadening the paradigm of PPD to include the language of trauma gives the suffering its due description, transforming the construct of postpartum depression itself.

How long have women waited to hear that PPD is traumatic, and survival a small miracle? How long have we known that untreated PPD is a war for women, from which some return wounded, others, not at all? If we take the leap and call it war, rather than a perinatal mood or anxiety disorder, its traumatic impact is validated in the eyes of society and science, giving childbearing women the modicum of respect and care a combat veteran might receive.

These experiences give me pause to consider the very nature of suffering of PPD itself, and the boundless capacity of the human spirit to grow because of it, or in spite of it. Acknowledging PPD as traumatic, we also acknowledge, then, that women have reactions to it that include trauma reactions. For clinicians, this acknowledgment could identify new methods of screening and intervention that includes trauma.

For researchers, this acknowledgment inspires new curiosity as to cross-disciplinary scholarship between trauma psychology and perinatal psychiatry. For families, the acknowledgment that PPD is traumatic offers new vocabulary to better describe and understand PPD. For providers, perhaps the connection between trauma and PPD will serve to push through barriers of stigma regarding maternal mental illness.

In essence, changing the language of PPD gives us the ability to understand it from multiple perspectives, to consider it from different ontological angles, and to know it intimately as a powerful component of the human condition.

CHANGING OWNERSHIP

One of the first written accounts of postpartum mood disorders was by Margery Kempe in 1436:

> *Wherefore after that, her child was born she, not trusting her life, sent for her ghostly father, as said before, in full will to be shriven of all her lifetime as near as she could. And, when she came to the point*

for to say that thing which she had so long concealed, her confessor was a little too hasty …and so she would no more say for nought he might do. And anon for dread she had of damnation on that one side and his sharp reproving on that other side, this creature went out of her mind and was wonderly vexed and labored with spirits half year eight weeks and odd days (as cited in Shannonhouse, 2003, p. 4).

Margery's honesty is indeed disarming and provides historical context to set the stage for future dialogue: perinatal mood and anxiety disorders have been around a long time. History shows us one other critical fact—childbearing and perinatal psychological disorders have been owned by male-dominated (and designed) professions, sciences, and medical systems given authority over birthing women.

Comparison to current models of maternity care reveals an alarming lack of evolution. A woman walking into a hospital to give birth today is still birthing according to the systems that own the knowledge about her body, her baby, and her wellness. Every protocol, from intake to discharge, is filtered through a system of care designed by institutions, not women. Her experience will not be hers, but regulated by preordained protocol of patient care. Similar, if not more restrictive, protocol rule psychiatric treatment facilities as well.

The institutions charged with psychiatric care demonstrate remain equally archaic. Look no further than the lack of mother-baby inpatient psychiatric programs in the United States. These specialized units allow mothers to room in with their babies during their stay.

When I wrote the first edition of this book, there were two inpatient psychiatric facilities in the United States. There are still only two: one in New York and the other in North Carolina. Without access to these units, mothers who require psychiatric

hospitalization for a postpartum mood or anxiety disorder are admitted to general population psychiatric facilities without access to their newborn baby. The rules remain that women are not considered the owners of their experience. Reproductive, physical, and mental health are owned by the experts, housed in clinical settings where experts have authority over anyone under their care.

I argue that where we go wrong is believing that this is the only way we can consider postpartum depression—through the expertise of authority. In our gut, we know women are the experts. Women who live and breathe the experience of a PMAD know more about their pain, and recovery, than medical manuals. The scientific research is helpful, yes. The novel theories, such as PPD as trauma, push the paradigm of maternal mental illness a bit. But in the end?

Perhaps the most necessary change we can make is this change of ownership. We cannot own the experiences of others. We don't own a mother's experience. She does. Simple as that.

FINAL THOUGHTS: RE-SEARCHING

Nearly two decades after my own PPD, my memories haven't faded. They are present and close, evidenced in my c-section scar, and the shape of my son's face even now as a man, looking like he did the night we met. Hindsight has provided no clarity; it haunts me.

This is a critical difference between my experience and those of the women in this book. I don't feel that I experienced transformation or posttraumatic growth as a result of my PPD. I got through it. Like so many of us, I got through it, but not without permanent damage. I lost precious parts of me in the process. I have since journeyed through whole decades of my life carrying the remnants of those months, lived on the edge of a bridge. Now, with 20 years later, I wonder if the journey through PPD ever really ends?

That question is where my next book begins.

REFERENCES

Abdollahi, F., & Zarghami, M. (2018). Effect of postpartum depression on women's mental and physical health four years after childbirth. *Eastern Mediterranean ealth ournal, 24*(10),1002.

Abebe, A., Tesfaw, G., Mulat, H., Hibdye, G., & Yohannes, K. (2019). Postpartum depression and associated factors among mothers in bahir dar town, northwest Ethiopia. *Annals of general psychiatry, 18.*

Abel, K. M., Hope, H., Swift, E., Parisi, R., Ashcroft, D. M. Kosidou, K., ... & Pierce, M. (2019). Prevalence of maternal mental illness among children and adolescents in the UK between 2005 and 2017: a national retrospective cohort analysis. *The lancet public health, 4*(6), e291-e300.

Abrams, L. S., Dornig, K., & Curran, L. (2009). Barriers to service use for postpartum depression symptoms among low-income ethnic minority mothers in the United States. *Qualitative health research, 19*(4), 535-551.

Accortt, E. E., Cheadle, A. C., & Schetter, C. D. (2015). Prenatal depression and adverse birth outcomes: an updated systematic review. *Maternal and child health journal, 19*(6), 1306-1337.

Agius, A., Xuereb, R. B., Carrick-Sen, D., Sultana, R., & Rankin, J. (2016). The co-existence of depression, anxiety and post-traumatic stress symptoms in the perinatal period: A systematic review. *Midwifery, 36,* 70-79.

Allens, N. B., & Badcock, P. B. (2003). The social risk hypothesis of depressed mood: Evolutionary, psychosocial, and neurobiological perspectives. *Psychological bulletin, 129*(6), 887.

Alloy, L. B., & Abramson, L. Y. (1979). Judgment of contingency in depressed and nondepressed students: Sadder but wiser? *Journal of experimental psychology: General, 108,* 441-485

Alloy, L. B., Albright, J. S., Abramson, L. Y., & Dykman, B.M. (1990). Depressive realism and non-depressive optimistic illusions: The role of the self. In R.E. Ingram (Ed.), *Contemporary psychological approaches to depression: Treatment, research, and theory* (pp. 71-86). Plenum Press.

American College of Obstetricians and Gynecologists Committee on Obstetric Practice. (2010). Committee opinion #453: Screening for depression during and after pregnancy. *Obstetrics & gynecology, 115*(2, Pt. 1), 394-395.

American College of Obstetricians and Gynecologists. (2010). *Your pregnancy and childbirth: month to month.* Retrieved from: https://www.acog.org/Clinical-Guidance-and-Publications/Your-Pregnancy-and-Childbirth-Month-to-Month.

American Psychiatric Association. (1994). *Diagnostic and statistical manual of mental disorders* (3rd ed.). Author.

American Psychiatric Association. (2000). *Diagnostic and statistical manual of mental disorders* (4th ed., Text rev.). Author.

American Psychiatric Association. (2013). *Diagnostic and statistical manual of mental disorders (DSM-5®).* American Psychiatric Pub.

Andrews, P. W., & Thomson, J. A., Jr. (2009). The bright side of being blue: Depression as an adaptation for analyzing complex problems. *Psychological review, 116*(3), 620-623.

Arroll, B., Goodyear-Smith, F., Crengle, S., Gunn, J., Kerse, N., Fishman, T., ... & Hatcher, S. (2010). Validation of PHQ-2 and PHQ-9 to screen for major depression in the primary care population. *The annals of family medicine, 8*(4), 348-353.

Atwood, M. (2012). *Dancing girls and other stories.* Random House.

Azad, R., Fahmi, R., Shrestha, S., Joshi, H., Hasan, M., Abdullah Nurus, S. K., . . . Sk, M. B. (2019). Prevalence and risk factors of postpartum depression within one year after birth in urban slums of Daka, Bangladesh. *PLoS One, 14*(5) https://dx.doi.org.tcsedsystem.idm.oclc.org/10.1371/journal.pone.02157

Azhari, A., Leck, W. Q., Gabrieli, G., Bizzego, A., Rigo, P., Setoh, P., ... & Esposito, G. (2019). Parenting stress undermines mother-child brain-to-brain synchrony: a hyperscanning study. *Scientific reports, 9*(1), 1-9.

Barkin, J. L., & Wisner, K. L. (2013). The role of maternal self-care in new motherhood. *Midwifery, 29*(9), 1050-1055.

Beck, A. T., & Steer, R. A. (1987). *BDI, Beck depression inventory: manual.* Psychological Corporation.

Beck, C., & Driscoll, J. (2006). *Postpartum mood and anxiety disorders: A clinician's guide.* Jones & Bartlett.

Beck, C., & Gable, R. K. (2000). Postpartum Depression Screening Scale: Development and psychometric testing. *Nursing Research, 49,* 272-282

Bell, L., Ham, J., Weinberg, M. K., Yergeau, E., & Tronick, E. (2004, May). In naturalistic home observations depressed mothers have a less positive and contingent relationship with their infants [Paper presentation]. *International Conference on Infant Studies:* Chicago, IL.

Bener, A., Gerber, L. M., & Sheikh, J. (2012). Prevalence of psychiatric disorders and associated risk factors in women during their postpartum period: A major public health problem and global comparison. *International journal of women's health, 4,* 191-200.

Bennett, W. L., Chang, H. Y., Levine, D. M., Wang, L., Neale, D., Werner, E. F., & Clark, J. M. (2014). Utilization of primary and obstetric care after medically complicated pregnancies: an analysis of medical claims data. *Journal of general internal medicine, 29*(4), 636-645.

Bennett, S., & Indman, P. (2019). *Beyond the blues: Understanding and treating prenatal and postpartum depression & anxiety* (4th Rev. ed.). Moodswings Press.

Berg, C., Callaghan, W. M., Syverson, C., & Henderson, Z. (2010). Pregnancy-related mortality in the United States: 1998 to 2005. *Obstetrics and gynecology, 116,* 1302-1309.

Bernstein, I. H., Rush, A. J., Yonkers, K., Carmody, T. J., Woo, A., McConnell, K., & Trivedi, M. H. (2008). Symptom features of postpartum depression: Are they distinct? *Depression and anxiety, 25,* 20-26.

Binder, E. B., Newport, D. J., Zach, E. B., Smith, A. K., Deveau, T. C., Altshuler, L. L., ... & Cubells, J. F. (2010). A serotonin transporter gene polymorphism predicts peripartum depressive symptoms in an at-risk psychiatric cohort. *Journal of psychiatric research, 44*(10), 640-646.

Bodnar-Deren, S., Klipstein, K., Fersh, M., Shemesh, E., & Howell, E. A. (2016). Suicidal ideation during the postpartum period. *Journal of women's health, 25*(12), 1219-1224.

Borra, C., Iacovou, M., & Sevilla, A. (2015). New evidence on breastfeeding and postpartum depression: the importance of understanding women's intentions. *Maternal and child health journal, 19*(4), 897-907.

Bowen, A., Stewart, N., Baetz, M., & Muhajarine, N. (2009). Antenatal depression in socially high-risk women in Canada. *Journal of epidemiology & community health, 63,* 414-416.

Bowlby, J. (1980). *Attachment and loss.* Basic Books.

Breslau, J., Kendler, K. S., Su, M., Gaxiola-Aguilar, S., & Kessler, R. C. (2005). Lifetime risk and persistence of psychiatric disorders across ethnic groups in the United States. *Psychological medicine, 35*(3), 317-327.

Bruce, F., Berg, C., Hornbrook, M., Whitlock, E., Callaghan, M., Bachman, D., . . . Dietz, P. (2008). Maternal morbidity rates in a managed care population. *Journal of obstetrics and gynecology, 111*(5), 1089-1095

Calhoun, L. G., & Tedeschi, R. G. (1990). Positive aspects of critical life problems: Recollections of grief. *Omega, 20,* 265-272.

Calhoun, L. G., & Tedeschi, R. G. (2004). The foundations of posttraumatic growth: New considerations. *Psychological inquiry, 15,* 93-102.

Campbell, S. B., Matestic, P., von Stauffenberg, C., Mohan, R., & Kirchner, T. (2007). Trajectories of maternal depressive symptoms, maternal sensitivity, and children's functioning at school entry. *Developmental psychology, 43,* 1202-1215.

Campbell, S. B., Morgan-Lopez, A. A., Cox, M. J., & McLoyd, V. C. (2009). A latent class analysis of maternal depressive symptoms over 12 years and offspring adjustment in adolescence. *Journal of abnormal psychology, 118,* 479-493.

Canady, R. B., Bullen, B. L., Holzman, C., Broman, C., & Tian, Y. (2008). Discrimination and symptoms of depression in pregnancy among African American and White women. *Women's health issues, 18*(4), 292–300.

Cents, R. A., Diamantopoulou, S., Hudziak, J. J., Jaddoe, V. W., Hofman, A. Verhulst, F. C., van den Berg, L., & Tiemeier, H. (2013). Trajectories of maternal depressive symptoms predict *child* problem behavior: The generation R study. *Psychological medicine, 43,* 13-25.

Chaudron, L., Kitzman, H. J., Peifer, K. L., Morrow, S., Perez, L. M., & Newman, M. C. (2005). Prevalence of maternal depressive symptoms in low-income Hispanic women. *Journal of clinical psychiatry, 66*(4), 418-423.

Chee, C. Y., Chong, Y. S., Ng, T. P., Lee, D. T., Tan, L. K., & Fones, C. S. (2008). The association between maternal depression and frequent non-routine visits to the infant's doctor—A cohort study. *Journal of affective disorders, 107*(1), 247-253.

Collado, M. A. O., Saez, M., Favrod, J., & Hatem, M. (2014). Antenatal psychosomatic programming to reduce postpartum depression risk and improve childbirth outcomes: a randomized controlled trial in Spain and France. *BMC pregnancy and childbirth, 14*(1), 22.

Cox, J. L., Holden, J. M., & Sagovsky, R. (1987). Detection of postnatal depression: Development of the 10-item Edinburgh postnatal depression scale. *British journal of psychiatry, 150,* 782-786.

Cox, E. Q., Sowa, N. A., Meltzer-Brody, S. E., & Gaynes, B. N. (2016). The perinatal depression treatment cascade: Baby steps toward improving outcomes. *The Journal of clinical psychiatry, 77*(9), 1189-1200

Curry, S. J., Krist, A. H., Owens, D. K., Barry, M. J., Caughey, A. B., Davidson, K. W., ... & Kubik, M. (2019). Interventions to prevent perinatal depression: US preventive services task force recommendation statement. *JAMA, 321*(6), 580-587.

Darwin, C. (1872). *The expression of the emotions in man and animals.* John Murray.

Davis, J. A., Alto, M. E., Oshri, A., Rogosch, F., Cicchetti, D., & Toth, S. L. (2020). The effect of maternal depression on mental representations and child negative affect. *Journal of affective disorders, 261*, 9-20.

Declerq, E. R., Sakala, C., Corry, M.P., Appelbaum, S., & Herrlich, A. (2013). *Listening to mothers^SM III: Pregnancy and childbirth.* Childbirth Connection.

Dikmen-Yildiz, P., Ayers, S., & Phillips, L. (2017). Depression, anxiety, PTSD and comorbidity in perinatal women in Turkey: A longitudinal population-based study. *Midwifery, 55*, 29-37.

Eaton, W. W., Smith, C., Ybarra, M., Muntaner, C., & Tien, A. (2004). Center for Epidemiologic Studies Depression Scale: review and revision (CESD and CESD-R).

Eberhard-Gran, M., Garthus-Niegel, S., Garthus-Nigel, K., &Eskild, A. (2010). Postnatal care: A cross-cultural and historical perspective. *Archives of women's mental health, 6,* 459-466.

eCouto, T. C., Brancaglion, M. Y. M., Alvim-Soares, A., Moreira, L., Garcia, F. D., Nicolato, R., ... & Corrêa, H. (2015). Postpartum depression: A systematic review of the genetics involved. *World journal of psychiatry, 5*(1), 103.

Eckerdal, P., Kollia, N., Löfblad, J., Hellgren, C., Karlsson, L., Högberg, U., ... & Skalkidou, A. (2016). Delineating the association between heavy postpartum hemorrhage and postpartum depression. *PLoS One, 11*(1), e0144274.

Elisei, S., Lucarini, E., Murgia, N., Ferranti, L., & Attademo, L. (2013). Perinatal depression: a study of prevalence and of risk and protective factors. *Psychiatr Danub, 25*(Suppl 2), S258-62.

Epstein, S. (1980). The self-concept: A review and the proposal of an integrated theory of personality. *Personality: Basic aspects and current research*, 81132.Faisal-Cury, A., & Menezes, P. R. (2019). Type of delivery is not associated with maternal depression. *Archives of women's mental health, 22*(5), 631-635.

Fawcett, E. J., Fairbrother, N., Cox, M. L., White, I. R., & Fawcett, J. M. (2019). The prevalence of anxiety disorders during pregnancy and the postpartum period: A multivariate Bayesian meta-analysis. *Journal of clinical psychiatry, 80*(4).

Fiala, A., Švancara, J., Klánová, J., & Kašpárek, T. (2017). Sociodemographic and delivery risk factors for developing postpartum depression in a sample of 3233 mothers from the Czech ELSPAC study. *BMC psychiatry, 17*(1), 104.

Figley, C. R. (1978). *Stress disorders among Vietnam veterans.* Brunner/Mazel.

Figueiredo, B., Dias, C. C., Brandão, S., Canário, C., & Nunes-Costa, R. (2013). Breastfeeding and postpartum depression: state of the art review. *Jornal de pediatria (versão em Português), 89*(4), 332-338.

Fisher, J., Cabral de Mello, M., Patel, V., Rahman, A., Tran, T., Holton, S., & Homes, W. (2012). Prevalence and determinants of common perinatal mental disorders in women in low- and lower-middle-income countries: A systematic review. *Bulletin of world health organization, 90*, 139-149G.

Gaillard, A., Le Strat, Y., Mandelbrot, L., Keita, H., & Dubertret, C. (2014). Predictors of postpartum depression: Prospective study of 264 women followed during pregnancy and postpartum. *Psychiatry research, 215*(2), 341-346.

Gan, Y., Xiong, R., Song, J., Xiong, X., Yu, F., Gao, W., ... & Zhang, J. (2019). The effect of perceived social support during early pregnancy on depressive symptoms at 6 weeks postpartum: a prospective study. *BMC psychiatry, 19*(1), 232.

Gavin, A., Tabb, K., Melville, J., Guo, Y., & Keaton, W. (2011). Prevalence and correlates of suicidal ideation during pregnancy. *Archive of women's mental health 14*, 239-246.

Gavin, N., Gaynes, B., Lohr, K., Meltzer-Brody, S., Garlehner, G., & Swinson, T. (2005). Perinatal depression: A systematic review of prevalence and incidence. *American journal of obstetrics and gynecology, 106*(5, Pt. 1), 1071-1083.

Gaynes, B., Gavin, N., Meltzer-Brody, S., Lohr, K., Swinson, T., Gartlehner, G., & Miller, W. (2005). *Perinatal depression: Prevalence, screening accuracy, and screening outcomes: Summary, evidence report, and technology assessment* (No. 119). Agency for Healthcare Research & Quality.

Gelabert, E., Gutierrez-Zotes, A., Navines, R., Labad, J., Puyané, M., Donadon, M. F., ... & Gratacós, M. (2019). The role of personality dimensions, depressive symptoms and other psychosocial variables in predicting postpartum suicidal ideation: a cohort study. *Archives of women's mental health*, 1-9.

Ghaedrahmati, M., Kazemi, A., Kheirabadi, G., Ebrahimi, A., & Bahrami, M. (2017). Postpartum depression risk factors: a narrative review. *Journal of education and health promotion, 6.*

Goodman, S. H., & Dimidjian, S. (2012). The developmental psychopathology of perinatal depression: Implications for psychosocial treatment development and delivery in pregnancy. *Canadian journal of psychiatry, 57*(9), 530-536.

Goodman, S. H., & Tully, E. C. (2009). Recurrence of depression during pregnancy: Psychosocial and personal functioning correlates. *Depression and anxiety, 26*(6), 557-567.

Guintivano, J., Sullivan, P. F., Stuebe, A. M., Penders, T., Thorp, J., Rubinow, D. R., & Meltzer-Brody, S. (2018). Adverse life events, psychiatric history, and biological predictors of postpartum depression in an ethnically diverse sample of postpartum women. *Psychological medicine, 48*(7), 1190-1200.

Hagen, E. H. (2011). Evolutionary theories of depression: a critical review. *Canadian journal of psychiatry. Revue Canadienne de psychiatrie, 56*(12), 716.

Halbreich, U., & Karkun, S. (2006). Cross-cultural and social diversity of prevalence of postpartum depression and depressive symptoms. *Journal of affective disorders, 91*(2-3), 97-111.

Hall, C. M., Molyneaux, E., Gordon, H., Trevillion, K., Moran, P., & Howard, L. M. (2019). The association between a history of self-harm and mental disorders in pregnancy. *Journal of affective disorders, 258*, 159-162.

Halligan, S. L., Murray, L., Martins, C., & Cooper, P. J. (2007). Maternal depression and psychiatric outcomes in adolescent offspring: A 13-year longitudinal study. *Journal of affective disorders, 97*(1), 145-154.

Hamdan, A., & Tamim, H. (2012). The relationship between postpartum depression and breastfeeding. *The International journal of psychiatry in medicine, 43*(3), 243-259.

Hammen, C. (2005). Stress and depression. *Annual review of clinical psychology, 1*, 293-319.

Hay, D. F., Pawlby, S., Waters, C. S., & Sharp, D. (2008). Antepartum and postpartum exposure to maternal depression: different effects on different adolescent outcomes. *Journal of p and psychiatry, 49*(10), 1079-1088.

Hecht, J. M. (2013). Stay: *A history of suicide and the philosophies against it.* Yale University Press.

Henshaw, C. (2007). Maternal suicide. In M. Pawson & J. Cockburn (Eds.), *Psychological challenges in obstetrics and gynecology: The clinical management* (pp. 157-164). Springer.

Holmes, T. H., & Rahe, R. H. (1967). The social readjustment rating scale. *Journal of psychosomatic research, 11,* 213-218.

Holzman, C., Eyster, J., Tiedje, L. B., Roman, L. A., Seagull, E., & Rahbar, M. H. (2006). A life course perspective on depressive symptoms in mid-pregnancy. *Journal of maternal & child health, 10*(2), 127-138.

Honikman, J. I. (2000). *Step by step: A guide to organizing a postpartum parent support network in your community.* Honikman.

Horowitz, M. (1976). *Stress response syndromes.* Jason Aronson.

Howard, L. M., Flach, C., Mehay, A., Sharp, D., & Tylee, A. (2011). The prevalence of suicidal ideation identified by the Edinburgh postnatal depression scale in postpartum women in primary care: Findings from the RESPOND trial. *BMC pregnancy & childbirth, 11,* 57.

Howard, L.M., Ryan, E.G., Trevillion, K., Anderson, F., Bick, D., Bye, A., Byford, S... & Demilew, J. (2018). Accuracy of the Whooley questions and the Edinburgh postnatal depression scale in identifying depression and other mental disorders in early pregnancy. *British journal of psychiatry 212,* 50–56.

Howard, L. M., Molyneaux, E., Dennis, C. L., Rochat, T., Stein, A., & Milgrom, J. (2014). Non-psychotic mental disorders in the perinatal period. *The Lancet, 384*(9956), 1775-1788.

Howell, E. A., Mora, P. A., Horowitz, C. R., & Leventhal, H. (2005). Racial and ethnic differences associated with early postpartum depressive symptoms. *Obstetrics and gynecology, 105,* 1442-1450.

Institute of Medicine. (2011, March 15). *Leading health indicators for healthy people 2020*: Letter report. Retrieved from https://iom.edu/Reports/2011/Leading-Health-Indicators-for-Healthy-People-2020.aspx

James, W. (1983). *Talks to teachers on psychology and to students on some of life's ideals* (Vol. 12). Harvard University Press.

Janoff Bulman, R., & Frieze, I. H. (1983). A theoretical perspective for understanding reactions to victimization. *Journal of social issues, 39*(2), 1-17.

Janoff-Bulman, R. (2011). *Shattered assumptions.* Simon and Schuster.

Jesse, D. E., & Swanson, M. S. (2007). Risks and resources associated with antepartum risk for depression among rural southern women. *Nursing research, 56*(6), 378-386.

Karraa, W. (2013). *Changing depression: A grounded theory of the transformational dimensions of postpartum depression.* ProQuest dissertations & theses global. (1494522311).

Karraa, W. (2014). *Transformed by postpartum depression: Women's stories of trauma and growth.* Praeclarus Press.

Katz, L. D. (2013). Pleasure. In N. Zalta (Ed.), *The Stanford encyclopedia of philosophy* (para. 1). Retrieved from https://plato.stanford.edu/archives/spr2013/entries/pleasure

Kempe, M. (2003). The book of Margery Kempe. In R. Shannonhouse (Ed.), *Out of her mind: Women writing on madness* (pp. 3-7). Modern Library. (Original work published 1436).

Kendall-Tackett, K. (2010). *Depression in new mothers: Causes, consequences, and treatment alternatives* (2nd ed.). Routledge.

Kimmel, M. C., Ferguson, E. H., Zerwas, S., Bulik, C. M., & Meltzer Brody, S. (2016). Obstetric and gynecologic problems associated with eating disorders. *International ournal of ating isorders, 49*(3), 260-275.

Knight, M. (2019). The findings of the MBRRACE-UK confidential enquiry into maternal deaths and morbidity. *Obstetrics, Gynaecology & reproductive medicine, 29*(1), 21-23.

Knitzer, J., Theberge, S., & Johnson, K. (2008). *Reducing maternal depression and its impact on young children: Toward a responsive early childhood policy framework.* National Center for Children in Poverty.

Ko, J. Y., Farr, S. L., Dietz, P. M., & Robbins, C. L. (2012). Depression and treatment among US pregnant and nonpregnant women of reproductive age, 2005–2009. *Journal of women's health, 21*(8), 830-836.

Kosidou, K., Dalman, C., Lundberg, M., Hallqvist, J., Isacsson, G., & Magnusson, C. (2011). Socioeconomic status and risk of psychological distress and depression in the Stockholm public health cohort: a population-based study. *Journal of affective disorders, 134*(1-3), 160-167.

Koutra, K., Vassilaki, M., Georgiou, V., Koutis, A., Bitsios, P., Kogevinas, M., & Chatzi, L. (2018). Pregnancy, perinatal and postpartum complications as determinants of postpartum depression: the Rhea mother–child cohort in Crete, Greece. *Epidemiology and psychiatric sciences, 27*(3), 244-255.

Kozhimannil, K. B., Trinacty, C. M., Busch, A. B., Huskamp, H. A., & Adams, A. S. (2011). Racial and ethnic disparities in postpartum depression care among low-income women. *Psychiatric services, 62*(6), 619-625.Kristof, N. D., & WuDunn, S. (2010). *Half the sky: Turning oppression into opportunity for women worldwide.* Vintage.

Kroenke, K., Spitzer, R., & Williams, J. (2001). The PHQ-9: Validity of a brief depression severity measure. *General internal medicine,16*(9), 606-613.

Kroenke, K., Spitzer, R. L., & Williams, J. B. (2003). The Patient health questionnaire-2: validity of a two-item depression screener. *Medical care,* 1284-1292.

Kumar, R. (1994). Postnatal mental illness: A transcultural perspective. *Social psychiatry and psychiatric epidemiology, 29,* 250-264.

Ladd, W. (2018). "Born out of fear": A grounded theory study of the stigma of bipolar disorder for new mothers. *The qualitative report, 23*(9), 2081-2104.

Lancaster, C. A., Gold, K. J., Flynn, H. A., Yoo, H., Marcus, S. M., & Davis, M. M. (2010). Risk factors for depressive symptoms during pregnancy: A systematic review. *American journal of obstetrics & gynecology, 202*(1), 5-14.

Lee, A. M., Lam, S. K., Mun Lau, S. M., Chong, C. S., Chui, H. W., & Fong, D. Y. (2007). Prevalence, course, and risk factors for antenatal anxiety and depression. *Obstetrics & gynecology, 110*(5), 1102-1112.

Leigh, B., & Milgrom, J. (2008). Risk factors for antenatal depression, postnatal depression and parenting stress. *BMH psychiatry, 8,* 11.

Letourneau, N., Salmani, M., & Duffett-Leger, L. (2010). Maternal depressive symptoms and parenting of children from birth to 12 years. *Western journal of nursing research, 32*(5), 662-685.

Letourneau, N. L., Tramonte, L., & Willms, J. D. (2013). Maternal depression, family functioning and children's longitudinal development. *Journal of pediatric nursing, 28*(3), 223-234.

Lewis, A. J. (1934). Melancholia: A clinical survey of depressive states. *British journal of psychiatry, 80*(329), 277-378.

Lewis, G. (2007). The Confidential enquiry into maternal and child health (CEMACH). *Saving Mothers' Lives*: reviewing *maternal deaths to make motherhood* safer–*2003–2005. The seventh report on confidential enquiries into maternal deaths in the United Kingdom.* CEMACH, 93.

Lindahl, V., Pearson, J., & Colpe, L. (2005). Prevalence of suicidality during pregnancy and postpartum. *Archive of women's mental health, 8*(2) 77-87.

Linley, P. A., & Joseph, S. (2004). Positive change processes following trauma and adversity. A review of the empirical literature. *Journal of traumatic stress, 17,* 11-12.

Liu, C. H., & Tronick, E. (2014). Prevalence and predictors of maternal postpartum depressed mood and anhedonia by race and ethnicity. *Epidemiology and psychiatric sciences, 23*(2), 201-209.

Luca, D. L., Garlow, N., & Statz, C. (2019). Societal costs of untreated perinatal mood and anxiety disorders in California. *Mathematica policy research, 4.*

Lucero, N. B., Beckstrand, R. L., Callister, L. C., & Sanchez Birkhead, A. C. (2012). Prevalence of postpartum depression among Hispanic immigrant women. *Journal of the american Academy of nurse practitioners, 24*(12), 726-734.

Maloney, J. (1952). Postpartum depression or third day depression following childbirth. *New Orleans child parent digest, 6,* 20-32.

Maloni, J. A., Przeworski, A., & Damato, E. G. (2013). Web recruitment and internet use and preferences reported by women with postpartum depression after pregnancy complications. *Archives of psychiatric nursing, 27*(2), 90-95.

Martini, A. (2006). *Hillbilly Gothic: a memoir of madness and motherhood.* Simon and Schuster.

Maslow, A. H. (1969). Toward a humanistic biology. *American psychologist, 24*(8), 724.

Mauri, M., Oppo, A., Borri, C., & Banti, S. (2012). Suicidality in the perinatal period: Comparison of two self-report instruments. Results from PND-ReScU. *Archives of women's mental health, 15*(1), 39-47.

McGuire, T. G., Alegria, M., Cook, B. L., Wells, K. B., & Zaslavsky, A. M. (2006). Implementing the Institute of Medicine definition of disparities: An application to mental health care. *Health services research, 41*(5), 1979-2005.

McNamara, J., Townsend, M. L., & Herbert, J. S. (2019). A systemic review of maternal wellbeing and its relationship with maternal fetal attachment and early postpartum bonding. *Plos one, 14*(7), e0220032.

Melville, J. L., Gavin, A., Guo, Y., Fan, M., & Katon, W. J. (2010). Depressive disorders during pregnancy: Prevalence and risk factors in a large urban sample. *Obstetrics and gynecology, 116*(5), 1064–1070.

Merrill, L., Mittal, L., Nicoloro, J., Caiozzo, C., Maciejewski, P. K., & Miller, L. J. (2015). Screening for bipolar disorder during pregnancy. *Archives of women's mental health, 18*(4), 579-583.

Miller, E. S., Hoxha, D., Wisner, K. L., & Gossett, D. R. (2015a). Obsessions and compulsions in postpartum women without obsessive compulsive disorder. *Journal of women's health, 24*(10), 825-830.

Miller, E. S., Hoxha, D., Wisner, K. L., & Gossett, D. R. (2015b). The impact of perinatal depression on the evolution of anxiety and obsessive-compulsive symptoms. *Archives of women's mental health, 18*(3), 457-461.

Moore, A. (2008). Hedonism. In N. Zalta (Ed.), *The Stanford encyclopedia of philosophy.*

Moore, M. T., & Fresco, D. M. (2007). Depressive realism and attributional style: Implications for individuals at risk for depression. *Behavior therapy, 38*, 144-154.

Mora, P. A., Bennett, I. M., Ito, I. T., Mathew, L., Coyne, J. C., & Culhane, J. F. (2009). Distinct trajectories of perinatal depressive symptomatology: Evidence from growth mixture modeling. *American journal of epidemiology, 169*(1), 24-32.

Morrison, T. (1973). *Sula.* Plume.

Mukherjee, S., Trepka, M. J., Pierre-victor, D., Bahelah, R., & Avnet, T. (2016). Racial/Ethnic disparities in antenatal depression in the united states: A systematic review. *Maternal and child health journal, 20*(9), 1780-1797.

Munk-Olsen, T., Ingstrup, K. G., Johannsen, B. M., & Liu, X. (2019). Population-based assessment of the recurrence risk of postpartum mental disorders: Will it happen again? *JAMA psychiatry.* https://doi:10.1001/jamapsychiatry.2019.3208

Murray, L., Arteche, A., Fearson, P., Halligan, S., Goodyer, I., & Cooper, P. (2011). Maternal postnatal depression and the development of depression in offspring up to 16 years of age. *Journal of the american academy of child & adolescent psychiatry, 50*(5), 460-470.

Murray, L., Cooper, P., Creswell, C., Schofield, E., & Sack, C. (2007). The effects of maternal social phobia on mother-infant interactions and infant social responsiveness. *Journal of child psychology and psychiatry, 48*(1), 45-52.

Myers, S., & Johns, S. E. (2018). Postnatal depression is associated with detrimental life-long and multi-generational impacts on relationship quality. *Peer journal, 6*, e4305.

National Institute of Mental Health. (November, 2017). *What is prevalence?* NIMH. https://www.nimh.nih.gov/health/statistics/what-is-prevalence.shtml#part_155620

Nadeem, E., Lange, J. M., Eddge, D., Fongwa, T., & Miranda, J. (2007). Does stigma keep poor young immigrant and U.S.-born Black and Latina women from seeking mental health care? *Psychiatric services, 58*, 1547-1554. https://doi:10.1176/appi.ps.58.12.1547

Nietzsche, F., & Crawford, C. (1997). The Dionysian worldview. *Journal of nietzsche studies*, 81-97.

Norhayati, M. N., Hazlina, N. N., Asrenee, A. R., & Emilin, W. W. (2015). Magnitude and risk factors for postpartum symptoms: a literature review. *Journal of affective disorders, 175*, 34-52.

Nunes-Cortez, M. A., Ferri, C. P., Manzolli, P., Soares, R. M., Drehmer, M., Buss, C., . . . Schmidt, M. (2010). Nutrition, mental health and violence: From pregnancy to postpartum cohort of women attending primary care units in Southern Brazil-ECCAGE study. *BMC psychiatry, 10*, 66.

Oakley, A. (1993). *Essays on women, medicine and health.* Edinburgh University Press.

Oates, M. (2003). Suicide: The leading cause of maternal death. *British journal of psychiatry, 183*, 279-281.

O'Donnell, M. J., Xavier, D., & Liu, L. (2010). Risk factors for ischemic and intracerebral hemorrhagic stroke in 22 countries (the interstroke study): A case control study. *The Lancet, 376*, 112-123.

O'Hara, M. W. (2009). Postpartum depression: What we know. *Journal of clinical psychology, 65*(12), 1258-1269.

O'Hara, M. W., & Segre, L. S. (2008). Psychological disorder of pregnancy and the postpartum. In R. S. Gibbs, B. Y. Karlan, A. F. Naey, & I. Nygaard (Eds.), *Danforth's obstetrics and gynecology* (10th ed.). Lippincott, Williams, & Wilkins.

O'Hara, M. W., & Wisner, K. L. (2014). Perinatal mental illness: definition, description and aetiology. *Best practice & research clinical obstetrics & gynaecology, 28*(1), 3-12.

O'Keane, V., Lightman, S., Patrick, K., Marsh, M., Papadopoulos, A. S., Pawlby, S., ... & Moore, R. (2011). Changes in the maternal hypothalamic pituitary adrenal axis during the early puerperium may be related to the postpartum 'blues'. *Journal of neuroendocrinology, 23*(11), 1149-1155.

Onah, M. N., Field, S., Bantjes, J., & Honikman, S. (2017). Perinatal suicidal ideation and behavior: psychiatry and adversity. *Archives of women's mental health, 20*(2), 321-331.

Oyston, C., Rueda-Clausen, C. F., & Baker, P. N. (2017). Current challenges in pregnancy-related mortality. *Obstetrics, gynaecology & reproductive medicine, 27*(7), 199-205.

Palladino, C. L., Singh, V., Campbell, J., Flynn, H., & Gold, K. J. (2011). Homicide and suicide during the perinatal period: Findings from the National Violent Death Reporting System. *Obstetrics & gynecology, 118*(5), 1056-1063.

Pan, A., Okereke, O. I., Sun, Q., Logroscino, G., Manson, J. E., Willett, W. C., ... & Rexrode, K. M. (2011). Depression and incident stroke in women. *Stroke, 42*(10), 2770-2775.

Paris, R., Bolton, R., Weinberg, M. (2009) Postpartum depression, suicidality, and mother-infant interactions. *Archives of women's mental health, 12*, 309–321

Pascoe, J. M., Stolfi, A., & Ormond, M. B. (2006). Correlates of mothers' persistent depressive symptoms: a national study. *Journal of pediatric health care, 20*, 261-269.

Patel, M., Bailey, R. K., Jabeen, S., Ali, S., Barker, N. C., & Osiezagha, K. (2012). Postpartum depression: A review. *Journal of health care for the poor and underserved, 23*, 534–542. https://dx.doi.org/10.1353/hpu.2012.0037

Perez-Rodriguez, M., Baca-Garcia, E., Oquendo, M., & Carlos, B. (2008). Ethnic differences in suicidal ideation and attempts. *Primary Psychiatry,15*, 44-58.

Prabhu, S., George, L. S., Shyamala, G., & Hebbar, S. (2019). Prevalence and associated risk factors of postnatal depression in South Asian region— systematic review. *Indian Journal of Public Health Research & Development, 10*(5), 329-333.

Priest, S. R., Austin, M. P., Barnett, B. B., & Buist, A. (2008). A psychosocial risk assessment model (PRAM) for use with pregnant and postpartum women in primary care settings. *Archives of women's mental health, 11*(5-6), 307.

Price, J., Gardner, R., & Wilson, D. R. (2007). Territory, rank, and mental health: The history of an idea. *Evolutionary psychology, 5*(3), 531-554.

Price, J., Sloman, L., & Gardner, R. (1994). The social competition hypothesis of depression. *British journal of psychiatry, 164*(3), 309-315.

Proietti, M., Pickston, A., Graffitti, F., Barrow, P., Kundys, D., Branciard, C., ... & Fedrizzi, A. (2019). Experimental test of local observer independence. *Science advances, 5*(9), eaaw9832.

Radloff, L. S. (1977). The CES-D scale: a self-report depression scale for research in the general population. *Applied psychological measurement, 1*: 385-401.

Reck, C., Struben, K., Backenstrass, M., Stefenelli, U., Reinig, K., Fuchs, T., ... & Mundt, C. (2008). Prevalence, onset and comorbidity of postpartum anxiety and depressive disorders. *Acta psychiatrica scandinavica, 118*(6), 459-468.

Records, K., & Rice, M. (2007). Psychosocial correlates of depression symptoms during the third trimester of pregnancy. *Journal of obstetric and gynecological nursing, 36*(3), 231-242.

Rich, A. (1995). *Of woman born: Motherhood as experience and institution.* WW Norton & Company

Rich-Edwards, J. W., Kleinman, K., Abrams, A., Harlow, B. L., McLaughlin, T. J., Joffe, H., & Gillman, M. W. (2006). Sociodemographic predictors of antenatal and postpartum depressive symptoms among women in a medical group practice. *Journal of epidemiology & community health, 60*(3), 221-227.

Richmond, E. (2019). Transformed by postpartum depression: Women's stories of trauma and growth. *Journal of prenatal & perinatal psychology & health, 33*(3), 251-253.

Riquin, E., Lamas, C., Nicolas, I., Lebigre, C. D., Curt, F., Cohen, H., ... & Godart, N. (2019). A key for perinatal depression early diagnosis: The body dissatisfaction. *Journal of affective disorders, 245*, 340-347.

Rosenberg, P. B., Mielke, M. M., Xue, Q. L., & Carlson, M. C. (2010). Depressive symptoms predict incident cognitive impairment in cognitive healthy older women. *American journal of geriatric psychiatry, 18*, 204-211.

Ross, L., & Dennis, C. (2009). The prevalence of postpartum depression among women with substance use, an abuse history, or chronic illness: a systematic review. *Journal of women's mental health, 18*(4), 475-486.

Ruddick, S. (1995). *Maternal thinking: Toward a politics of peace.* Beacon Press.

Rumi, J. (2004). *The essential Rumi: New expanded edition* (C. Barks, Trans.). Harper One. (Original work published 1995)

Saczynski, J. S., Beiser, A., Seshardi, S., Auerbach, S., Wolf, P. A., & Au, R. (2010). Depressive symptoms and risk of dementia: The Framingham heart study. *Neurology, 75*, 35-41.

Sahrakorpi, N., Koivusalo, S. B., Eriksson, J. G., Kautiainen, H., Stach-lempinen, B., & Roine, R. P. (2017). Perceived financial satisfaction, health related quality of life and depressive symptoms in early pregnancy. *Maternal and child health journal, 21*(7), 1493-1499.

Sarah, S. B., Forozan, S. P., & Leila, D. (2017). The relationship between model of delivery and postpartum depression. *Annals of tropical medicine and public health, 10*(4), 874.

Schnatz, P. F., Nudy, M., Shively, C. A., Powell, A., & O'Sullivan, D. M. (2011). A prospective analysis of the association between cardiovascular disease and depression in middle-aged women. *Menopause, 18*(10), 1096-1100.

Segre, L. S., O'Hara, M. W., Arndt, S., & Stuart, S. (2007). The prevalence of postpartum depression: The relative significance of three social status indices. *Social psychiatry & psychiatric epidemiology, 42*, 316-321.

Segre, L. S., O'Hara, M. W. & Losch, M. E. (2006). Race/ethnicity and perinatal depressed mood. *Journal of reproductive & infant psychology* 24(2), 99-106.

Seligman, M. (1975). *Helplessness: On depression, development, and death.* W. H. Freeman.

Seligman, M., & Csikszentmihalyi, M. (2000). Positive psychology: An introduction. *American psychologist, 55*(1), 5-14. https://doi:10.1037//0003-66X.55.1.5

Sharifzadeh, M., Navininezhad, M., & Keramat, A. (2018). Investigating the relationship between self-esteem and postpartum blues among delivered women. *Journal of research in medical and dental sciences, 6*(3), 357-362.

Sharma, V., Xie, B., Campbell, M. K., Penava, D., Hampson, E., Mazmanian, D., & Pope, C. J. (2014). A prospective study of diagnostic conversion of major depressive disorder to bipolar disorder in pregnancy and postpartum. *Bipolar disorders, 16*(1), 16-21.

Shellman, L., Beckstrand, R. L., Callister, L. C., Luthy, K. E., & Freeborn, D. (2014). Postpartum depression in immigrant Hispanic women: A comparative community sample. *Journal of the American association of nurse practitioners, 26*(9), 488-497.

Shi, P., Ren, H., Li, H., & Dai, Q. (2018). Maternal depression and suicide at immediate prenatal and early postpartum periods and psychosocial risk factors. *Psychiatry research, 261*, 298-306.

Sichel, D., & Driscoll, J. W. (2000). *Women's moods, women's minds: what every woman must know about hormones, the brain, and emotional health.* Quill.

Simmons, L. A., Huddleston-Casas, C. A. & Berry, A. (2007). Low-income rural women and depression: Factors associated with self-reporting. *American journal of health behavior, 31*, 657-666.

Slomian, J., Honvo, G., Emonts, P., Reginster, J. Y., & Bruyère, O. (2019). Consequences of maternal postpartum depression: A systematic review of maternal and infant outcomes. *Women's health, 15*, 1745506519844044.

Snyder, C. R., & Lopez, S. J. (Eds.). (2002). *Handbook of positive psychology.* Oxford University Press.

Spitzer, R., Kroenke, K., & Williams, J. (1999). Validation and utility of a self-report version of Prime-MD: The PHQ primary-care study. Primary care evaluation of mental disorders. Patient Health Questionnaire. *JAMA, 282*(18), 1737-1744.

Stein, A., Pearson, R.M., Goodman, S.H., Rapa, E., Rahman, A., McCallum, M., Howard, L.M., Pariante, C.M. (2014). Effects of perinatal mental disorders on the fetus and child. *The Lancet 384,* 1800–1819.

Stockman, J. K., Hayashi, H., & Campbell, J. C. (2015). Intimate partner violence and its health impact on ethnic minority women. *Journal of women's health, 24*(1), 62-79.

Taylor, R. E., & Kuo, B. C. (2019). Black American psychological help-seeking intention: An integrated literature review with recommendations for clinical practice. *Journal of psychotherapy integration, 29*(4), 325.

Tambağ, H., Turan, Z., Tolun, S., & Can, R. (2018). Perceived social support and depression levels of women in the postpartum period in Hatay, Turkey. *Nigerian journal of clinical practice, 21*(11), 1525-1530.

Tedeschi, R. G. & Calhoun, L. G. (1995). *Trauma and transformation: Growing in the aftermath of suffering.* Sage.

Tedeschi, R. G., & Calhoun, L. G. (1996). The posttraumatic growth inventory: Measuring the positive legacy of trauma. *Journal of traumatic stress, 9,* 455-471.

Tedeschi, R. G., & Calhoun, L. G. (2004). Posttraumatic growth: Conceptual foundations and empirical evidence. *Psychological inquiry, 15*(1), 1-18.

Tedeschi, R. G., & Calhoun, L. G. (2006). Expert companions: Posttraumatic growth in clinical practice. In *Handbook of posttraumatic growth: Research and practice* (pp. 291-310). Erlbaum.

Tedeschi, R. G., & Calhoun, L. G. (2008). Beyond the concept of recovery: Growth and the experience of loss. *Death studies, 32,* 27-39.

Tennants, C. (2002). Life events, stress, and depression: A review of recent findings. *Australian and New Zealand journal of psychiatry, 36*(2), 173-182.

Thoreau, H. D. (2006). *Walden.* Yale University Press.

Trevathan, W. (2010). *Ancient bodies, modern lives: How evolution has shaped women's health.* Oxford University Press.

Triplett, K. N., Tedeschi, R. G., Cann, A., Calhoun, L. G., & Reeve, C. L. (2012). Posttraumatic growth, meaning in life, and life satisfaction in response to trauma: *Psychological trauma: theory, research, practice, and policy, 4*(4), 400-410.

Ukatu, N., Clare, C. A., & Brulja, M. (2018). Postpartum depression screening tools: a review. *Psychosomatics, 59*(3), 211-219.

U.S. Centers for Disease Control. (2008). *Prevalence of self-reported postpartum depressive symptoms in 17 states, 2004-2005. MMWR Morbidity and Mortality Weekly Report, 57*(14), 361-366.

U.S. Centers for Disease Control. (2009). *HIV Surveillance Report, 21.* Retrieved from https://www.cdc.gov/hiv/topics/surveillance/resources/reports

U.S. Centers for Disease Control. (2013). Depression surveillance data sources. Retrieved from https://www.cdc.gov/mentalhealth/data_stats/depression.htm

Vaezi, A., Soojoodi, F., Banihashemi, A. T., & Nojomi, M. (2019). The association between social support and postpartum depression in women: A cross sectional study. *Women and birth, 32*(2), e238-e242.

Vesga-Lopez, O., Blanco, C., Keyes, K., Olfson, M., Grant, B., & Hasin, D. (2008). Psychiatric disorders in pregnant and postpartum women in the United States. *Archives of general psychiatry, 65,* 805-815.

Wang, P. S., Berglund, P., Olfson, M., Pincus, H. A., Wells, K. B., & Kessler, R. C. (2005). Failure and delay in initial treatment contact after first onset of mental disorders in the National Comorbidity Survey Replication. *Archives of general psychiatry, 62*(6), 603.

Westdahl, C., Milan, S., Magriples, U., Kershaw, T., Rising, S., & Ickovics, J. (2007). Social support and social conflict as predictors of prenatal depression. *Obstetrics and gynecology, 110*(1), 134-140.

Wilson, R. S., Hoganson, G. M., Rajan, K. B., Barnes, L. L., Mendes de Leon, C. F., & Evans, D. A. (2010). Temporal course of depressive symptoms during the development of Alzheimer's disease. *Neurology, 75,* 21-26.

Wint, D. (2011). Depression: A shared risk factor for cardiovascular and Alzheimer's disease. *Cleveland clinical journal of medicine, 78*(Suppl.1), S44-S46.

Wisner, K., Logsdon, M. C., & Shanahan, B. R. (2008). Web-based education for postpartum depression: Conceptual development and impact. *Archives of women's mental health,11*(5-6), 377-385.

Wisner, K., Perel, J., Findling, R., & Hinnes, R. (2001). Prevention of recurrent postpartum depression: A randomized clinical trial. *Journal of clinical psychiatry, 62*(2), 82-86.

Wisner, K., Perel, J., Peindl, K. S., & Hanusa, B. H. (2004). Timing of depression recurrence in the first year after birth. *Journal of Affective Disorders, 78*, 249-252. https://doi:10.1016/S0165-0327(02)00305-1

Wisner, K., Sit, D. Y., McShea, M. C., Rizzo, D. M., Zoretich, R. A., Hughes, C. L., . . . Hanusa, B. H. (2013). Onset timing, thoughts of self-harm, and diagnoses in postpartum women with screen-positive depression findings. *Journal of the American medical association/psychiatry, 70*(5), 490-498. https://doi:10.1001/jamapsychiatry.2013.87

Witt, W., DeLeire, T., Hagen, E., Wichmann, M., Wisk, L., Spear, H., . . . Hampton, J. (2010). The prevalence and determinants of antepartum mental health problems among women in the USA: A nationally representative population-based study. *Archives of women's mental health, 13*, 425-437.

Woolf, V. (2014). *A room of one's own (1929).* In the People, Place, and Space Reader (pp. 338-342). Routledge.

World Health Organization. (1992). *The ICD-10 classification of mental and behavioral disorders: Clinical descriptions and diagnostic guidelines.* Author.

Wszołek, K., Żak, E., Żurawska, J., Olszewska, J., Pięta, B., & Bojar, I. (2018). Influence of socio-economic factors on emotional changes during the postnatal period. *Ann agric environ med, 25*(1), 41-45.

Wu, Z., Zhao, P., Long, Z., Li, J., Yang, G., Zhang, Q., ... & Li, H. (2019). Biomarker screening for antenatal depression in women who underwent caesarean section: a matched observational study with plasma lipidomics. *BMC psychiatry, 19*(1), 259.

Zaidi, F., Nigam, A., Anjum, R., & Agarwalla, R. (2017). Postpartum depression in women: a risk factor analysis. *Journal of clinical and diagnostic research: JCDR, 11*(8), QC13.

Zhong, Q. Y., Gelaye, B., Miller, M., Fricchione, G. L., Cai, T., Johnson, P. A., ... & Williams, M. A. (2016). Suicidal behavior-related hospitalizations among pregnant women in the USA, 2006–2012. *Archives of women's mental health, 19*(3), 463-472.

APPENDIX

THE CHANGING DEPRESSION SURVEY

In 2014, I conducted an informal, anonymous online survey in order to collect more data regarding suicidality during untreated PPD and women's perceptions of key support figures in accessing help for PPD. Recruitment via social media for women who have suffered from postpartum depression has been supported in the methodological literature (Maloniet al., 2013). Recruitment was done anonymously through social media advertisement, setting an audience target to recruit women who are over the age 20 and English-speaking. I collected data via a secured, online statistical analytical service, between October 2013 and January 2014. The service maintains confidentiality and provides tracking to block repeat entries. Demographic data included age, employment, and time elapsed since the episode of PPD had occurred.

AGE

The majority of respondents (n = 300; 61.7%) were between the ages 30-39; 19.1% (n = 93) were between the ages 21-29; and 15.0% (n = 73) were ages 40-49 (see Table 2).

EMPLOYMENT

35.4% (n=172) of respondents reported being employed and working 1-39 hours per week. 29.8% (n=145) reported being employed and working more than 40 hours a week. 28.4% (n =

138) reported not being employed and not looking for work. 4.3% (n = 21) reported not being employed and currently looking for work, and 10 respondents (2.1%) reported being disabled. No respondents (0.0%) reported being retired.

TIME ELAPSED SINCE PPD

Four hundred and eighty-three of the 486 responded to this question. The majority, 56.9% (n = 275) reported it had been 0-2 years since they had experienced PPD; 25.9% (n =125) responded 2-5 years since they had experienced PPD; 12.2% (n = 59) reported 5-10 years since they had experienced PPD; and 38 (7.9%) respondents reported over 10 years since they had experienced PPD.

Which category below includes your age?		
Answer Options	Response Percent	Response Count
17 or younger	0.0%	0
18-20	0.8%	4
21-29	19.1%	93
30-39	61.7%	300
40-49	15.0%	73
50-59	3.3%	16
60 or older	0.0%	0
	answered questions	486

Table 2: Age Range - Changing Depression Survey

SUICIDALITY

With a total response of 486, significant data trends emerged. I asked two questions regarding suicidality in the survey: (a) Do you consider your experience of postpartum depression (PPD) to have been life-threatening and (b) Did you experience thoughts of harming yourself or others during postpartum depression (PPD)? The question, *Do you consider your experience of postpartum depression (PPD) to have been life-threatening?* had a total of 486 completed responses, with 58.8% (n = 286) responding "no" and 41.2% (n = 200) responding "yes." Figure 5 represents these findings.

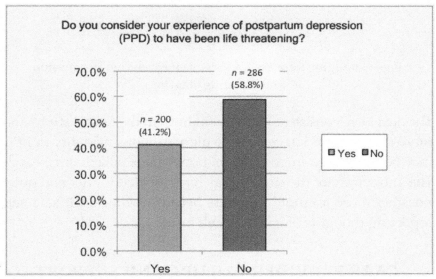

Fig 5: Changing Depression Survey - PPD as Life-Threatening

The second question, *did you experience thoughts of harming yourself or others during postpartum depression (PPD)?* was completed by all 486 respondents. 61% (n = 297) responded "yes" while 38.9% (n =189) responded "no." Figure 6 represents those findings.

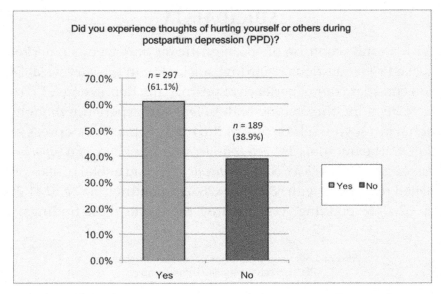

Fig 6: Changing Depression Survey - Postpartum Depression and Harming Ideation

The data were consistent with my findings in the formal study, and more importantly, suggested the high level of suicidality in PPD may be overlooked in postpartum populations polled for research. The anonymity of the survey may have yielded higher and quite possibly more accurate numbers because women felt safe self-reporting thoughts of harming self or others.

CARE PROVIDER FAILURE AND SUPPORT

Two questions in the Changing Depression Survey addressed who respondents felt were most and least helpful in getting them help for PPD. The first question, *who was MOST responsible for your getting help for postpartum depression (PPD)?* yielded data regarding women's perception of self as an agent in accessing care for PPD.

Given six options (see Figure 7), 65.4% (n= 318) selected "Self"; 23.0% (n = 112) selected "Partner"; 16.9% (n = 82) selected "Family Member"; 11.7% (n = 57) selected "Medical Care Provider"; 8.8% (n = 55) selected "Other (Friend),"and 6.6% (n =32) selected "Therapist." Figure 7 represents the findings.

When asked, who was LEAST helpful in getting you help for postpartum depression (PPD), the majority of women (n= 210; 43.2%) reported Medical Care Providers (OB/GYN, Midwife, General, or Family Physician) as least helpful; 21% (n=105) reported family members as least helpful; 20.6% (n=100) reported that their partner was least helpful; 19.3 % (n=93) reported Self as least helpful, and 6.8% (n=33) reported therapist as least helpful (see Figure 8).

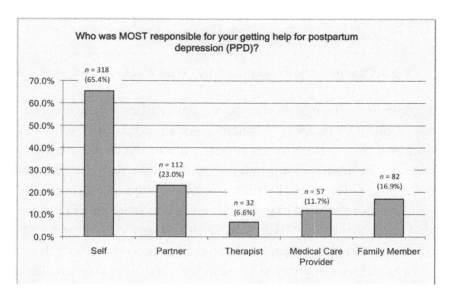

Fig 7: Changing Depression Survey - Who Was Most Helpful?

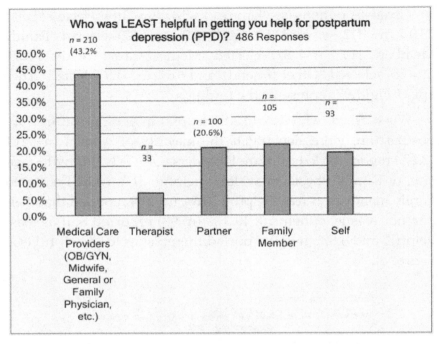

Fig 8: Changing Depression Survey - Who Was Least Helpful?

The data in my formal study and the data gathered here suggest a lack of provider support in helping women who suffer with PPD. Moreover, in contrast to the reports of women experiencing deficiencies in help-seeking behaviors, this data strongly suggests the opposite. The majority of women (n = 318) reported that they were the most helpful in getting themselves help for PPD. Again, what are we missing? The gaps in direct service from provider to patient and the lack of understanding as to the strength and resourcefulness of women present interesting opportunities to review standard practices of care and research the inner potential of women who experience mood or anxiety disorders postpartum.

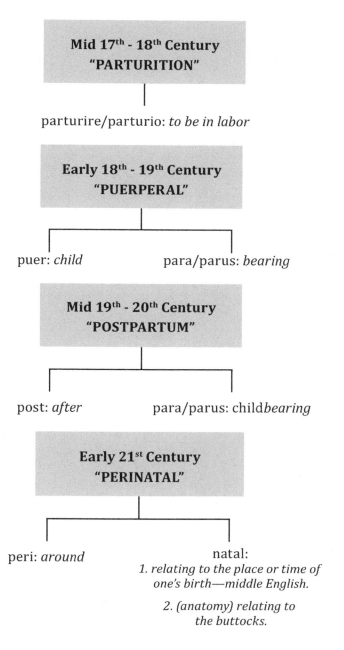

Fig 9: Timing and Language (Ladd, 2020)

Made in the USA
Las Vegas, NV
25 July 2021